Diabetes
BURNOUT
What to Do When You Can't Take It Anymore

WILLIAM H. POLONSKY, PhD, CDE

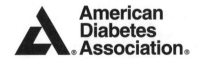

American Diabetes Association

Book Acquisitions, Robert J. Anthony; Editor, Aime M. Ballard; Production Director, Carolyn R. Segree; Production Manager, Peggy M. Rote; Composition, Harlowe Typography, Inc.; Text and Cover Design, Wickham and Associates, Inc.; Printer, Transcontinental Printing, Inc.

Printed in Canada
3 5 7 9 10 8 6 4

The suggestions and information contained in this publication are generally consistent with the Clinical Practice Recommendations and other policies of the American Diabetes Association, but they do not represent the policy or position of the Association or any of its boards or committees. Reasonable steps have been taken to ensure the accuracy of the information presented. However, the American Diabetes Association cannot ensure the safety or efficacy of any product or service described in this publication. Individuals are advised to consult a physician or other appropriate health care professional before undertaking any diet or exercise program or taking any medication referred to in this publication. Professionals must use and apply their own professional judgment, experience, and training and should not rely solely on the information contained in this publication before prescribing any diet, exercise, or medication. The American Diabetes Association—its officers, directors, employees, volunteers, and members— assumes no responsibility or liability for personal or other injury, loss, or damage that may result from the suggestions or information in this publication.

∞ The paper in this publication meets the requirements of the ANSI Standard Z39.48-1992 (permanence of paper).

ADA titles may be purchased for business or promotional use or for special sales. To purchase this book in large quantities, or for custom editions of this book with your logo, contact Lee Romano Sequeira, Special Sales & Promotions, at the address below, or at LRomano@diabetes.org or 703-299-2046.

American Diabetes Association
1701 North Beauregard Street
Alexandria, Virginia 22311

Chapters 5, 11, and 14 are based on articles that the author wrote previously for Diabetes Self-Management magazine.

Library of Congress Cataloging-in-Publication Data
Polonsky, William H., 1952–
    Diabetes burnout: what to do when you can't take it anymore / William H. Polonsky.
        p. cm.
    Includes index.
    ISBN 1-580-40033-7 (pbk.)
    1. Diabetes—Popular works. 2. Diabetes—Psychological aspects. I. Title.
RC660.4.P66 1999   99-044735

Contents

Foreword

I cheered when I was invited to write the foreword for *Diabetes Burnout: What to Do When You Can't Take It Anymore*, by my friend and colleague Dr. William Polonsky. Bill was the first psychologist ever to hold a position on the staff of the Joslin Diabetes Center in Boston. And I was fortunate to be the second psychologist at Joslin and to work closely with Bill there for about 7 years. Bill was my introduction to a personal/professional "champion" for people with diabetes. He has long been an advocate for individuals coping with diabetes and has helped all of us understand more clearly the many struggles that this chronic disease imposes on children, adults, and their families.

In *Diabetes Burnout*, Bill guides us toward a broad range of solutions for the complexities of living with diabetes. There are other books available that urge individuals and families who live with diabetes to "take charge" of, to "live well" with, and to "outsmart" the disease. These guides send the clear message that if only one has the "right" knowledge, skills, tools, and attitudes, then life with diabetes can be a smooth journey. In contrast, Bill introduces a quite different and more reality-based message. He acknowledges that the medical prescriptions to follow a meal plan, manage blood sugar levels, or integrate diabetes tasks into the family can never be carried out perfectly. In his commitment to people with diabetes, Bill speaks out about the truth that living with diabetes means sometimes dealing with discouragement, aggravation, and despair. From the first chapter to the last, he encourages the reader to be realistic rather than perfectionistic. And he supports this breakaway approach both with research and with touching, sometimes humorous stories, voices of the many individuals with diabetes whom he has helped.

I am particularly pleased that a consistent theme throughout *Diabetes Burnout* is that families matter. Through the stories of Warren, Robert, and Sarah, Bill illustrates the delicate balance between support and supervision in families living with diabetes. He clarifies how family members can learn to be constructively involved in diabetes management and to keep caring from becoming criticizing.

I am enthusiastic about this book for patients and their families, as well as for the professionals who care for them. *Diabetes Burnout: What to Do When You Can't Take It Anymore* is an engaging book, written with wisdom, humor, and thoughtfulness about navigating the potholes and bumps that are always along the journey of life with diabetes.

Barbara J. Anderson, PhD
Senior Psychologist, Joslin Diabetes Center
Associate Professor, Department of Psychiatry
Harvard Medical School

Acknowledgments

Whilе writing this book, I was fortunate to have the generous support of many friends and colleagues. They took the time to provide me with expert guidance, critical feedback, and careful review of many of the chapters. My thanks to Ron Ray, Katie Davis, Linda Gonder-Frederick, Rich Jackson, Tom Conant, and Jim Warram. I am also thankful for the warm and wise counsel I have received over the years from my esteemed colleagues in the field of behavioral diabetes—including Barbara Anderson, Richard Rubin, Dan Cox, and John Zrebiec.

In truth, the most important contributors to this book are the innumerable patients with diabetes who honored me with their trust and with their stories. It has been a great privilege to learn from you all.

Finally, I am most deeply indebted to Reegan Ray, who cajoled me along in every stage of this process and continues to guide and support me every day. Without her wisdom, patience, and love, this book would never have happened. Thanks, Reeg!

Introduction

Is diabetes driving you crazy? If so, welcome to the club! In fact, a very large club! It has been my honor and pleasure to meet many thousands of people with diabetes over the years, and almost all of them are battling in some way or another with the illness. Some are infuriated with diabetes, some depressed. Others are frightened, frustrated, guilt-ridden, or in denial. Underlying all of these different emotions is something very important, a common psychological struggle that I never quite knew how to describe or explain—until I met Howard, a young man who had been living with type 1 diabetes for most of his life. Howard had been at war with the disease since his early teenage years. In our very first meeting, he summed up his feelings about diabetes in a clear and concise manner: "Diabetes sucks!"

Howard pinpointed for me how many of my patients really felt. Living with diabetes can be terribly frustrating and difficult. It is not just a simple matter of eating right or taking your medications properly. Diabetes is often an emotional struggle as well. Indeed, addressing and overcoming the emotional stresses of diabetes may be one of the most important steps you can take to manage the illness successfully. Unfortunately, it is too easy for both patients and doctors to neglect this personal side of the illness.

Like many others, Howard was suffering from *diabetes burnout*. Burnout is what happens when you feel overwhelmed by diabetes and by the frustrating burden of diabetes self-care. People who have burned out realize that good diabetes care is important for their health, but they just don't have the motivation to do it. At a fundamental level, they are at war with their diabetes—and they are losing.

Are you battling with diabetes burnout? Do any of the following sound familiar?

- Feeling overwhelmed and defeated by your diabetes.
- Feeling angry about diabetes, feeling frustrated by the self-care regimen, and/or having other strong, negative feelings about diabetes.
- Feeling that diabetes is controlling (or trying to control) your life.
- Worrying that you are not taking care of your diabetes well enough and yet feeling unable, unmotivated, or unwilling to change.
- Telling yourself that diabetes management is not important, that complications can't happen to you, and yet not being able to escape a sense of impending doom.
- Partially or fully "quitting" your diabetes care, thinking about diabetes as little as possible, and telling yourself that living with high blood sugars is not a problem.
- Avoiding any and all diabetes-related tasks that might give you feedback about the consequences of your poor self-care (for example, blood glucose monitoring or doctor visits).

■ Feeling alone with your diabetes, perhaps because you are feeling so ashamed about diabetes that you keep it a secret from everyone.

The more of these items that accurately describe you, the more likely it is that you have burned out on diabetes.

As you will see, diabetes burnout is understandable, but in the long term, it is a destructive and deadly way of coping with diabetes. If you are feeling burned out, there are three important things you need to know:

1. You are not alone (diabetes burnout is quite common).
2. You are not a bad person (given the pressures and the disappointments associated with living with diabetes, burnout is understandable).
3. Your situation is far from hopeless (burnout can be conquered).

This book has been written especially for you who are feeling burned out by diabetes and for those who love you. It examines how the stresses of diabetes can build, how diabetes burnout occurs, and most importantly, *how burnout can be overcome*. So let's get started!

The Personal Side of Diabetes

CHAPTER 1
On the Road to Diabetes Burnout

From the outside, diabetes looks like it should be fairly simple. After all, all you have to do is take your insulin or oral medications every day at the right time and in the right amount, eat perfectly without ever "cheating," check your blood glucose regularly, and exercise frequently. Balance these tasks with each other so that your blood glucose levels never get too low or too high. And don't gain—or lose—too much weight. Stay vigilant at all times just in case something goes wrong. Finally, remember that you must continue to do all of this every day for the rest of your life, with no vacations from diabetes, ever! Wow.

Living with diabetes is not easy at all. No matter how much attention and effort you are able to give to your diabetes care, you can be certain that something will eventually go wrong. There will be crazy days when blood glucose levels rise or fall dramatically *for no apparent reason.* There will be frustrating days when you just can't stop eating. And there may be scary days when minor—or major—complications suddenly appear.

Joan Williams Hoover is a well-known author in diabetes who first developed the concept of diabetes burnout.

In an article for physicians, she describes how diabetes can require a great deal of personal effort and a large number of personal decisions every day. Most importantly, she writes:

> And even the constant need for decisions might be tolerable, if only the results were predictable. Few things generate burnout like the awful frustration of having followed instructions and done everything just right and still be failing to get the diabetes into control. At those times it seems no use to continue to try. Think how discouraging it is to fail at something you really wanted to do. Then consider what it must feel like to have diabetes and be failing at something you never, ever, wanted to do in the first place.

Given all of the work, responsibility, decisions, and at least occasional disappointment, it is remarkable that anyone is able to manage diabetes successfully year after year. There are some people who do. However, for many others, the frustrations of diabetes can become overwhelming, leading to feelings of helplessness, depression, or even worse. Let's meet some of these folks.

MEL'S STORY

When I met Mel, he was 29 years old. He was a hardworking carpenter who had been living with type 1 diabetes for 18 years. As a teenager, Mel and his parents had often battled about his diabetes care. His parents had demanded that he manage his diabetes very carefully, but they never really offered any help. They insisted that "you learn to take care of it by yourself." During his high school years, Mel began to feel more and more irritated and burdened by the demands of diabetes, especially because he wanted to "fit in" with his schoolmates. He fought more and more frequently with his parents. And he began to feel that there was just no good reason to go along with their demands for better self-care.

Since high school, Mel had mostly ignored his diabetes, though he had always taken his insulin regularly. He had never followed any type of meal plan. And he tended to eat large amounts of chocolate and other sweets every day. He checked his blood glucose about once every month or so ("Why bother checking more? It's always high," he told me). And he almost never saw a doctor. None of his friends knew that he had diabetes, and Mel himself did his best to think about it as little as possible. Although he insisted that diabetes was "no big deal," Mel had become increasingly worried about the possibility of long-term complications. And although he didn't like talking about it, Mel admitted that he had always been angry about his diabetes and that he had felt overwhelmed and defeated by the illness for many years.

LOIS'S STORY

Lois was a 54-year-old administrator for a local school system. She had been diagnosed with type 2 diabetes when she was 48. Frightened by the possibility of long-term complications, she had always been anxious to manage her diabetes well. She told me that she had been relatively successful in the first months following diagnosis, but she soon became overwhelmed and frustrated. The hospital dietitian had recommended a highly structured meal plan that required Lois to give up many of her favorite foods. As the months wore on, this new way of eating felt more and more restrictive. Following her doctor's advice, Lois had also tried to begin a regular walking schedule. However, the demands of her job soon made this too difficult to follow. Despite Lois's best efforts over those first few months, she was unable to lose weight and had experienced several frightening episodes of mild hypoglycemia (low blood glucose).

Not surprisingly, Lois's attempts at self-management had slowly deteriorated. By the time we met, she was continuing to take her oral medication faithfully each day, but she was checking her blood glucose only rarely. She was following her prescribed meal plan, but only through the daylight hours. By dinnertime, Lois would begin to binge on cookies and crackers, and this would continue unchecked until bedtime. She had not taken a brisk walk or done any serious exercise in years. Her husband and close friends were worried about her health and were constantly pushing her to "try harder." But this had not been helpful. It had only increased her sense of isolation with diabetes. Lois tried not to think about her illness and avoided seeing her physician, who she feared would recommend that she begin taking insulin. When she did allow herself to think about diabetes, she felt angry and frustrated with herself.

REGINA'S STORY

Regina was a 19-year-old college student. As she described it to me, she had been "at war" with diabetes ever since she was diagnosed at age 12. Regina came from a cold and violent home. Her parents were so busy fighting with each other that there was little time available to help Regina manage her diabetes. Her blood glucose control was very poor. She averaged one or two admissions for diabetic ketoacidosis (DKA) each year.

Regina had lived on her own for the past 2 years, and her poor diabetes self-management had only worsened. Her doctor had prescribed a regimen that included long-acting (ultralente) and short-acting (regular) insulins. However, Regina had not taken any ultralente in over a year. And she only took regular insulin, typically in very large amounts, every several days when she suspected that DKA was approaching. Regina had not tested her blood glucose in several years. She was obese and was preoccupied with losing weight. She felt unable to control her eating, which included multiple episodes of bingeing each day and occasional vomiting.

Regina felt ashamed about her behavior and frightened that long-term complications would affect her soon. She was angry at her diabetes and angry at her physician (whom she saw as blaming and uncaring). She felt depressed and hopeless. Regina was anxious to change, but she feared that any attempt at better blood glucose control would lead to even greater weight gain.

SAM'S STORY

Sam was 66 years old and a successful businessman. He had been living with type 2 diabetes for 3 years. Despite pleas from his family and physician, Sam saw little reason to make any changes in his lifestyle for diabetes. He did not mind taking his oral medications each day. However, he saw no point in adjusting his eating or being less sedentary. Sam's blood glucose levels were consistently above 250 mg/dl, and his cholesterol and blood pressure were both dangerously high. But this did not seem important to him. As he explained it to me, "What's the difference? We're all going to die anyway!"

Sam's wife, who was worried sick about him, would argue with him constantly. She urged him to stop eating so many sweets, to start exercising, and to see his doctor more regularly. But none of this had any effect on Sam. Many years earlier, Sam had seen his father die from complications caused by diabetes. He was certain that this was to be his fate as well. In his heart, Sam felt doomed by the illness. The diagnosis had been a death sentence. And Sam believed that there was nothing he could do to alter his own fate.

BURNOUT IS COMMON

There are many, many people with stories similar to those of Mel, Lois, Regina, and Sam. They are male and female, young and old, new to diabetes and veterans of the disease. They are not bad, stupid, or weak people. They are normal folks who are struggling with diabetes for understandable reasons. And their struggles take many shapes. Many feel out of control and overwhelmed by their diabetes. They feel helpless that things can ever improve. Some feel alone with their diabetes. Others battle with denial, never truly accepting the reality of diabetes in their lives. And what they all have in common is diabetes burnout.

BURNOUT AND POOR SELF-CARE

Even though there has been such positive news over the past few years about the great benefits of good self-care, diabetes self-care seems to be growing worse and worse. Research evidence now clearly shows that blood glucose management and other healthy actions can dramatically lower your risk of long-term complications. But, as can be seen from the statistics in the box "News about Diabetes Self-Care," many people are not taking advantage of this opportunity to ensure a longer and healthier life for themselves. This is not because they lack willpower or are stupid. Instead, the major culprit is diabetes burnout. Why? Because burnout saps your motivation to take care of yourself. And not taking care of yourself can lead to long-term complications such as eye, kidney, or heart disease.

THE JOB OF DIABETES

Consider this analogy. Have you ever known anyone who had a frustrating job in which he or she worked harder and harder each day, yet it seemed that his or her actions didn't make any real difference? For example, a nurse on a cancer ward works hard for the patients every day. Despite her efforts and caring, she has not received a raise in many years, her supervisors and colleagues never congratulate her on the great work she is doing, and many of her patients continue to worsen and die. Over time, these stresses begin to take their toll. The nurse may end up feeling helpless, chronically overextended and depleted, inadequate, and guilty that she is somehow failing at her job. These are the core features of burnout.

Living with diabetes can be a very similar kind of "job," especially if you begin to feel that the day-to-day effort needed to manage diabetes is too burdensome and frustrating and the results not good enough to make the effort worthwhile. Much like the nurse suffering from job burnout, the person with diabetes burnout may feel very mixed up about whether he wants to continue his "job."

NEWS ABOUT DIABETES SELF-CARE

Here are some statistics that may surprise you:

1. Problems with blood glucose monitoring
   - In a nationwide survey, 21% of patients with type 1 diabetes reported that they never checked their blood glucose levels. Never! Of those patients with type 2 diabetes using insulin, 41% never monitored. Of those with type 2 who were not using insulin, 76% reported that they never monitored.
   - In recent surveys at the Joslin Diabetes Center and two large clinics in California, my colleagues and I found that 21–25% of patients rarely or never followed their doctor's recommendations for blood glucose monitoring. In a recent nationwide survey, 12% of patients reported rarely or never following recommendations for checking their blood glucose levels.
2. Problems with healthy eating
   - In recent surveys, 10–24% of patients with diabetes reported that they rarely or never follow their health care team's dietary recommendations.
   - In our Joslin survey, 22% of patients reported knowing that they were supposed to follow a certain meal plan, but they felt that it was usually or always impossible to do so.
   - A study of a well-known diabetes education program showed that the program greatly helped patients to begin eating better and exercising more. However, when contacted 1 year later, most patients had returned to their old, less healthy habits.
3. Problems with regular exercise
   - In recent national surveys, 31–38% of patients with diabetes reported that they rarely or never follow their health care team's recommendations for regular exercise.
   - In our recent surveys of patients with diabetes, my colleagues and I found that 37–43% of patients *never* exercise. Only 38% managed to exercise three times per week or more.

News about Diabetes Self-Care *(continued)*

4. Problems with diabetes medications
   ▪ A series of studies have found that many women with type 1 diabetes (somewhere between 10% and 40%, depending on the study) regularly take less than the prescribed amount of insulin. One new study also suggests that some patients take less than the prescribed amount of their oral diabetes medications.

He may hate diabetes and believe that it controls his life, yet he knows that he cannot quit. He may even become preoccupied with worry about diabetes, while at the same time doing as little as possible.

THE CHALLENGE OF BURNOUT

In my own practice, I have met far too many people who, because of diabetes burnout, have chosen to ignore their diabetes for years or, in some cases, decades. Tragically, many have been hit hard by long-term complications— eye disease, kidney disease, heart disease, painful nerve damage, amputations, and more. The arrival of serious complications is sometimes a wake-up call for taking charge of one's diabetes management, but not always. Diabetes burnout is so powerful that it can persist even in the face of complications.

However, diabetes burnout is *not* invincible. The good news is that it can be defeated. All of the people who you have met in this chapter—Mel, Lois, Regina, and Sam— have overcome burnout and have made peace with diabetes. They are successfully managing their blood glucose levels. And they are living healthy and satisfying lives. You can, too!

CHAPTER 2
The Real Story about Motivation in Diabetes: Recognizing and Overcoming Barriers

Why is diabetes self-care so difficult for so many people? If you are struggling with unhealthy eating habits, a reluctance to monitor your blood glucose, or some other self-care problem, what is really keeping you from managing your diabetes more successfully? Many people, including a large number of health care providers, believe that the explanation is a lack of self-discipline, too little willpower, stupidity, or "denial." In other words, they think you are just not trying hard enough.

But there is little scientific evidence to support these beliefs. People who are managing their diabetes poorly do not necessarily have a problem with self-discipline or willpower. And there is no evidence that those with poor self-care are less frightened about long-term complications than anyone else. Indeed, our research has shown the opposite to be true: Those with the poorest self-management are often more frightened about complications than those with better self-care. It is easy to accuse someone of "not having enough willpower" or "not accepting their diabetes," but that is usually unfair and inaccurate. For many people, the real reason for poor self-management is diabetes burnout.

WHO ISN'T MOTIVATED?

To truly understand burnout, we must consider three truths about motivation and diabetes care.

1. No one is unmotivated to take care of his or her diabetes. No one. Instead, they are perfectly motivated to do just what they are doing—and that's the problem. For example, Mrs. Smith has not followed her doctor's request that she exercise (specifically, that she go for a walk after dinner each evening). She is not unmotivated to go walking. She likes the idea of exercise very much. However, she is more strongly motivated to do what she has always done: watch "Wheel of Fortune" and "Jeopardy," her favorite TV shows, instead! The important point here is that no one, neither you nor anyone else, is in need of a "motivation transplant." Rather, you need to understand the unique pressures that make it hard for you to take care of diabetes.

2. There are many long-term benefits to taking care of diabetes, but not very many immediate ones. For every interesting decision that needs to be made ("Should I eat that lovely piece of cake?"), we think first about short-term consequences ("That's going to taste really good!") and then—to a lesser extent—about long-term consequences ("If I keep eating so many sweets, I'm likely to have higher blood glucose levels and this increases my risks for complications"). Unfortunately, the decisions most human beings make are more strongly influenced by their thoughts about short-term results than by their thoughts about long-term results. In fact, short-term consequences are so powerful that they can cause us to change our behavior and our attitudes without even realizing that we're doing so. Unfortunately, in a disease like diabetes, the most important benefits are not immediate (in particular, the prevention of long-term complications), whereas there can be immediate, positive consequences for ignoring diabetes concerns ("This cake tastes terrific!"). So it is easy to see how short-term influences could lead to a loss of interest in diabetes self-care.

3. No one feels motivated to do something if the costs seem to outweigh the benefits. There are costs and benefits, pros and cons, for every possible diabetes self-care action, whether it be eating healthfully, checking your blood glucose, or making time for exercise. You make self-care decisions—often without knowing it—on the basis of your beliefs about those costs and benefits. If it seems to you that the benefits clearly outweigh the costs, managing diabetes will feel relatively easy. However, if you see diabetes care as being such a burden that it outweighs the potential benefits, then it may seem completely reasonable to try and ignore your diabetes. So diabetes burnout is more likely to occur when you believe the costs of taking good care of diabetes outweigh any possible benefits.

Even if you know that there are several powerful benefits to taking good care of diabetes, the barriers to good self-management can often seem enormous. It is important to take a good, hard look at the benefits of and the barriers to effective diabetes care.

THE BENEFITS OF GOOD CARE

The two major benefits of effective diabetes management are

■ a positive impact on long-term complications: a healthier and more vibrant life for the future

■ a positive impact on short-term complications: a healthier and more vibrant life almost immediately

If you lower your blood glucose levels, you also lower the possibility that long-term complications will develop. And even a relatively small improvement in average blood glucose levels toward the normal range can have an enormous influence on long-term health. Perfection is not necessary. Even a small improvement in blood glucose can lead to significant health benefits.

In the short-term, high blood glucose levels can make you feel tired, irritable, and moody. You may have more frequent skin infections, and wounds may heal more slowly or not at all. The evidence is clear that when you can lower high blood sugars, remarkable changes begin to occur rapidly. People report more energy, better mood, and even better sleep. An additional benefit is that better blood glucose management means fewer visits to the emergency room and fewer hospital stays. So if good diabetes care can dramatically improve the quality of your life both now and in the future, it would seem reasonable to conclude that it must be worth the effort to manage diabetes as carefully as possible.

But Knowledge Is Not Enough

In 1992, the results from the Diabetes Control and Complications Trial (DCCT) were announced to the world. This study presented the first conclusive evidence that careful management of blood glucose has strikingly beneficial effects. Many of the major American diabetes centers believed that their clinics would soon be crowded with patients demanding the help and guidance needed to achieve good diabetes management. To prepare for this, new switchboards were purchased and extra receptionists were hired. But what happened? Well, nothing happened. Few calls were received, and the new switchboards were soon dismantled. How could this be? The moral of the story seems to be that becoming aware of major health benefits is not really a powerful motivator for most people.

As an analogy, consider the benefits of quitting smoking. Most Americans are well aware that smoking is bad for them. But very few smokers have ever picked up a packet of cigarettes, read the warning label, and concluded: "Lung cancer? Heart disease? Oh my goodness, I think I'll stop smoking immediately!" Warning labels have been placed on cigarette products and advertising for many decades. So if becoming aware of the benefits was that important, most smokers would have stopped long ago. One of the problems seems to be that most people don't really understand how much smoking increases the likelihood of pain and misery in their future or how much quitting smoking will improve their long-term health.

Similarly, knowing what is good for them may not be enough to inspire people to take care of their diabetes. What might be holding them back?

THE BARRIERS TO GOOD SELF-CARE

Although you may be aware of the benefits of good self-care, the many *barriers* to good care can have a more powerful influence on your feelings and actions. The barriers are like straws on the proverbial camel's back. If there are only a few, you may be able to overcome these pressures and still manage diabetes successfully. One barrier too many, however, and the camel's back collapses, leading to compromises in your self-care and eventually to diabetes burnout. There are so many possible barriers to good diabetes management that it is useful to divide them into three categories: personal, interpersonal, and environmental. Let's take a look at some of the barriers you might meet in each of these categories.

Personal Barriers

Your own thoughts, feelings, and attitudes can make diabetes management difficult. This category includes depression, coping styles, eating disorders, knowledge, beliefs, feelings, fears, and expectations.

Chronic Depression

When you're feeling very blue, it can be hard to summon up any energy to care about your diabetes. In particular, chronic and severe depression can make even the simple tasks of daily life seem too difficult to accomplish. Worse yet, long-term high blood glucose levels, which can result from poor management, can deepen depression, leading to an ever-worsening downward spiral.

Poor Coping Styles

Everyone has a characteristic way of responding to difficult situations. Some people deal with stress by *thinking*: They

---

PERSONAL BARRIERS

1. Chronic depression
2. Poor coping styles
3. Eating disorders
4. Lack of knowledge about diabetes
5. Inaccurate health beliefs
6. Negative feelings about diabetes
7. Fear of hypoglycemia
8. Fear and frustration about weight gain
9. Unrealistic or unclear expectations about self-care

---

seek to understand what is wrong, devise solutions, and take action to overcome the problem. Others respond primarily by *feeling*: They start with an emotional response, such as anger or disappointment, and then devise a way to handle their feelings (perhaps by exercising briskly or trying to think about other things).

There is good scientific evidence that those who respond to the trials and tribulations of diabetes with mostly a feeling approach tend to manage their diabetes less effectively. Imagine, for example, the aggravation of checking your blood glucose and discovering that it is surprisingly high. The best response is to focus on resolving the problem ("Okay, what should I do about this high number?")—in other words, to use a thinking approach. Instead, if your response is a feeling approach ("Oh no, I've done something terribly wrong, I hate myself"), you are unlikely to take effective action to deal with the high blood glucose.

Eating Disorders

There are many ways in which people battle with food and with their body images. These include clinical disorders such as *bulimia nervosa* and *anorexia nervosa*, as well as problems such as binge eating and emotional eating. Eating disorders are heartbreakingly common. And for most people, eating is by far the biggest battle in diabetes care. Any eating disorder can interfere with your ability to follow a healthy meal plan and can make good diabetes management all but impossible.

Lack of Knowledge about Diabetes

Not having the skills and knowledge to manage diabetes is, of course, a serious obstacle to good care. Tragically, many people with diabetes have never received any formal training in diabetes and don't know enough about their illness. They have not learned how to follow a healthy meal plan, how to exercise safely, how to check their blood glucose, how to examine their feet, or how to use blood glucose readings to adjust their medication, exercise, or eating.

Inaccurate Health Beliefs

Two health beliefs in particular can be barriers to good care. Many people believe that diabetes is not a serious disease or that they will not develop diabetes complications. If they believe that good diabetes management will not have an effect on their health, they are unlikely to make much of an effort. On the other hand, many people believe that diabetes is so terrifying and serious that there is no hope. Often, these are the people who have seen their parents or other loved ones damaged and destroyed by diabetes. They feel that they are also doomed to suffer the most terrible complications and there is nothing they can do about it. From this perspective, good diabetes management is again meaningless.

It is important to realize that both of these extreme beliefs are wrong. Developing more accurate health beliefs—diabetes *is* serious, but you are not doomed—can help you handle the fear and other emotions that may surface when you think about the possibility of long-term complications.

Negative Feelings about Diabetes

Many people have developed a terrible relationship with their diabetes. They feel at war with the illness. They feel that they are in an ongoing battle to determine whether diabetes will control them or whether they will control diabetes. They feel overwhelmed and frequently helpless. So they try to think about diabetes as little as possible. Feelings of hatred, anger, fear, sadness, and guilt are common. Of course, all of these feelings lie at the heart of diabetes burnout. And it is easy to see how such feelings could interfere with your desire and ability to manage diabetes as effectively as possible.

Fear of Hypoglycemia (Low Blood Glucose)

Because good diabetes management usually brings high blood glucose levels closer to the normal range, there may be some risk of your blood glucose dropping too low. This is especially true if you are taking insulin or certain oral hypoglycemic (blood glucose–lowering) medications. If you are already nervous about low blood glucose (perhaps you have had a scary, embarrassing, or unpleasant experience with hypoglycemia in the past), then you may be uncomfortable with the idea of improving your diabetes care. Such fears are common and reasonable. And they can influence your feelings about diabetes care even if you are not aware of them.

Fear and Frustration about Weight Gain

When you achieve better control of your blood glucose, you may gain weight. For many people, an increase of even 10–20 pounds is not unusual. If you are someone who is concerned about your shape and weight, a significant weight gain can be a very disheartening consequence of good self-care. Why bother working so hard, you may wonder, when relaxing your self-care efforts may help you to manage your weight more successfully (even if it does raise your blood glucose)?

Unrealistic or Unclear Expectations about Self-Care

Many people have become convinced that they must manage their diabetes perfectly. They believe that they must follow a healthy and balanced meal plan without ever straying from it, that they must rigidly adhere to an exercise plan, that they must check their blood glucose and take medications on a tight and unbending schedule, and that their blood glucose must always be in the normal range. This is not only overwhelming and exhausting, it is also impossible. Thus, if you feel that you must be perfect with your diabetes care, you will end up feeling like a failure. And this can make you feel like quitting diabetes care altogether.

Similarly, people who are not certain about their diabetes care goals may also lose interest in good care. For example, what does it mean to be successful with your meal plan? If you ate a plateful of cookies only one night during the past week, rather than your usual seven nights, is that success? If you cannot determine at the end of the day or week whether or not you are doing a good job with your diabetes care, then it is hard to give yourself the positive support and feedback that you need to stay on track.

Interpersonal Barriers

Your relationships with other people can affect your diabetes management. This category includes family conflict, support issues, confusion about care responsibilities, the "doormat" syndrome, and your relationship with your doctor.

INTERPERSONAL BARRIERS

1. Family conflict
2. Too little support
3. Too much support
4. Family confusion about self-care responsibilities
5. The "doormat" syndrome
6. A poor relationship with your doctor

Family Conflict

For everyone with diabetes—children, teens, and adults—self-management is poorer when there are high levels of stress in the family. Frequent arguments, hostility, and feelings of alienation among family members can influence the moods and actions of everyone. In a home atmosphere like this, your diabetes management can become just one more opportunity (or excuse) for an argument. Not surprisingly, you may lose interest in good self-care.

Too Little Support

Living with diabetes can be lonely. Many people have no one in their lives that they can really talk to about living with this tough illness. Even those who do have friends and close family members may discover that these loved ones are often uninterested or unsupportive when it comes to self-management efforts. In some cases, friends and family may not recognize the need for moral support ("Look, if you would just stop eating the cookies I buy for the kids, this would really be no big deal"). In other cases, whether they know it or not, friends or family may be actively working against self-management efforts ("C'mon, one little piece isn't going to hurt you!"). There can be no doubt that the stresses of living with diabetes are much more likely to wear you down when you have little or no emotional support from others.

Too Much Support

Many people have friends and family members who want to help them take care of their diabetes, *whether they like it or not*. It is not uncommon for loved ones to act like "diabetes police." They tell you what to do and work hard to provide you with much more help in managing your diabetes than you actually want. They may offer suggestions such as, "You shouldn't be eating that" or "You seem upset; maybe you should check your blood sugar." Unfortunately, a nasty battle for personal independence may then take place. The more your friends and family act like diabetes police, the more likely you may be to do just the opposite—you may start to behave like a "diabetes criminal."

Family Confusion about Self-Care Responsibilities

A major barrier to good diabetes self-management is a lack of clear agreement regarding who exactly is responsible for each of the many self-management tasks. For example, is your spouse responsible for whether or not you follow a healthy meal plan? Is the child with diabetes responsible for remembering when to check his blood glucose? There is no right or wrong answer. However, when there is no clarity among family members, this becomes a fertile breeding ground for conflict. In such an environment, it becomes easy for the person with diabetes to feel either abandoned or overly controlled. In all such cases, self-management is likely to suffer.

The "Doormat" Syndrome

Many people dedicate their lives to caring for others, especially for their families. Unfortunately, some of these nurturing souls may become so focused on caring for their loved ones that they put their own needs on the very bottom of the list. They become, in essence, "doormats" for their families. And this is a difficult habit to break. If this person develops diabetes, he or she may be reluctant to begin making the small or large household changes needed for successful self-management. For example, consider the case of Mrs. Dunn. She knows that it is too hard to avoid eating cookies when they are so easily available in her own kitchen, but she doesn't want to inconvenience her spouse or children by suggesting that cookies no longer be purchased. Until she speaks up about her need to eat fewer cookies and allows her family to support her, her diabetes management efforts will not be successful.

A Poor Relationship with Your Doctor

If you don't have a good working relationship with your doctor, then it is unlikely that you will get the guidance, support, and feedback that you need to manage your diabetes successfully over the years. And, unfortunately, frustrations with doctors are far from rare. Many people complain that their doctors don't give them clear enough directions on how to manage diabetes, don't spend enough time with them, don't take their concerns seriously enough, or unfairly blame them for "cheating" or not trying hard enough. To be fair, the doctors may not be the only ones at fault. For example, some people who are angry about having diabetes tend to take that anger out on their doctors.

Environmental Barriers

Your environment can also have a negative effect on diabetes self-management. This category includes stress, priorities, finances, and scheduling problems.

ENVIRONMENTAL BARRIERS

1. Chronic life stress
2. Competing priorities
3. Financial burdens of diabetes care
4. An unstructured life

Chronic Life Stress

If you have personal problems at work and at home, financial worries, or time pressures, it may be more difficult to take the time for self-care. Also, for some people with diabetes, chronic stress may lead to hormonal changes that affect blood sugars directly.

Competing Priorities

Diabetes self-management tasks may not get done when you have too many other demands in your life. These can include the demands of special occasions, like shopping and cooking for the holiday season, or everyday demands, like driving the children to and from their activities or coping with a deadline at work. When you feel overwhelmed by other priorities, you may feel you just don't have the time for self-care.

Financial Burdens of Diabetes Care

Diabetes care can be expensive. Your diabetes management might be more successful if you were using a different medication or an insulin pump, or were checking your blood glucose more frequently. A meeting with a diabetes specialist might be helpful. Participation in a diabetes education program is likely to be of enormous benefit. However, when your insurance does not cover these expenses and your own income is limited, it may feel necessary to cut corners.

An Unstructured Life

If you are in college, retired, unemployed, or working as a homemaker, you may be relatively flexible in terms of your daily schedule. However, without the regular structure provided by a job or some other schedule, it can be difficult to remember when to take medications, to check blood glucose on a regular basis, or to make time for exercise. Following a healthy meal plan may be especially difficult. When much of your free time is spent at home—dangerously close to your kitchen—you may have a hard time stopping yourself from snacking too often.

CONQUERING BURNOUT

You can see why day-to-day diabetes care is difficult for so many people and why there are so many cases of diabetes burnout. Even though the benefits to good self-care are well-proven, the obstacles—personal, interpersonal, and environmental—are so numerous that it can be easy to convince yourself that good care is just not worth the effort. The cons often seem to outweigh the pros.

The list of self-care barriers presented above is far from complete, but even this short list gives you a sense of the obstacles you may face. It may seem impossible, but you can make it over or around every single one of these barriers. The first step is to take a good, hard look at your own, often unconscious, barriers to better diabetes management. You may have already started to do that as you looked at the lists in this chapter. In the next chapter, you will assemble a list of your own personal obstacles and prepare a plan for action.

CHAPTER 3
Preparing for Action

Do you wonder whether you are struggling with diabetes burnout? Do you have a good sense of how distressing diabetes really is for you? Complete Worksheet 3.1 to find out.

Once you have completed the worksheet, break out your calculator and add up your responses to determine your total score. In case you are concerned about your mathematical abilities, remember that your total score must be a number between 6 and 36. Record your score below:

On Worksheet 3.1, my total score was _____.

So what does your score mean? How distressed by diabetes are you?

▊ **Not distressed.** If your total score is 6–12, congratulations! Compared to most people, the degree to which you are aggravated about your diabetes is fairly low. Approximately one-half of all the people who have been surveyed to date (which included people with type 1 and type 2 diabetes) fall within this category. In fact, many people (24%) actually had a very low score of 6, indicating that *none* of these six issues were worrisome for them.

WORKSHEET 3.1: HOW BURNED OUT ARE YOU?

Directions: In day-to-day life, there may be numerous problems and hassles concerning diabetes and they can vary greatly in severity. Problems may range from minor hassles to major life difficulties. Listed below are several potential problem areas that people with diabetes may experience. Consider the degree to which each of the items may have distressed or bothered you *during the past month* and circle the appropriate number.

Please note that we are asking you to indicate the degree to which each item may be bothering you in your life, NOT whether the item is merely true for you. If you feel that a particular item is not a bother or problem, you would circle 1. If it is very bothersome, you would circle 6.

	Not a problem		Moderate problem		Serious problem	
1. Feeling that diabetes is taking up too much of my mental and physical energy every day.	1	2	3	4	5	6
2. Feeling "burned out" by the constant effort to manage diabetes.	1	2	3	4	5	6
3. Feeling that I am often failing with my diabetes regimen.	1	2	3	4	5	6
4. Feeling that diabetes controls my life.	1	2	3	4	5	6
5. Not feeling motivated to keep up my diabetes self-management.	1	2	3	4	5	6
6. Feeling overwhelmed by my diabetes regimen.	1	2	3	4	5	6

- **Moderately distressed.** A total score of 13–20 is somewhat higher than average, indicating that you are feeling more miserable about your diabetes than do most people.
- **Very distressed.** If your total score is 21–26, your emotional battle with diabetes is pretty serious. There is a good likelihood that you are struggling with diabetes burnout.
- **Extremely distressed.** If your score is 27 or higher, there can be little doubt that you are at war with your diabetes. Scores this high are rare; of the patients who have been surveyed to date, only about 4% fall in this range. Diabetes burnout is all but certain.

DISCOVERING YOUR PERSONAL OBSTACLES

Regardless of your total score, you are likely to find some new ideas, emotional support, or other benefits in this book. However, the book is especially targeted to those who fall into one of the three distressed ranges, and especially those of you who scored 21 and above. As overwhelmed as you may feel, the good news is that your emotional battle with diabetes can be ended. You can make peace with diabetes.

The first step is to investigate what it is about diabetes that is driving you crazy. This probably makes the most sense to those of you in the "not distressed" and "moderately distressed" categories. Yes, you may say, there certainly are areas of diabetes that I find more burdensome or worrisome than others. However, to those of you in the "very distressed" and "extremely distressed" categories, the idea behind this investigation may seem odd. After all, you may be thinking, I know what is aggravating about my diabetes—everything! But let's examine this more carefully:

In chapter 2, three types of diabetes barriers were introduced—personal, interpersonal, and environmental. In addition, there are the daily demands of diabetes care, which can also be quite burdensome. Thus, there are four major factors that can contribute to feeling overwhelmed by diabetes:

■ **your day-to-day struggle with diabetes self-care** (how well, or how poorly, you are coping with self-care tasks)

■ **your social relationships** (the degree to which you do, or don't, have others in your life who are rooting for you and supporting your efforts)

■ **your own attitudes and feelings** (the degree to which you are, or are not, burdened by emotional problems and by destructive beliefs about diabetes)

■ **your environmental stresses** (how well, or how poorly, you are coping with the broad stresses of life and with the unique stresses of diabetes problems)

Which of these four factors are important for you? You can find out right now by completing Worksheet 3.2.

Once you have completed the worksheet, add up your responses to items 1–8 to determine your
SELF-CARE SCORE: _____.
Add up your responses to items 9–16 to determine your
SOCIAL SCORE: _____.
Add up your responses to items 17–24 to determine your
FEELINGS SCORE: _____.
And add up your responses to items 25–32 to determine your STRESS SCORE: _____.

You can begin to interpret your scores by using the three simple rules that follow:

1. Any of the four scores that is greater than 16 is likely to represent a problem area for you.
2. The highest of the four scores is probably your most difficult problem area.
3. A score that is less than 16 suggests that this is not a problem area for you. In fact, this particular area may be one of your strengths.

To apply these rules, please complete Worksheet 3.3 now.

If you study your responses to Worksheet 3.3, you can see that not everything is driving you crazy (at least for most of you), and you can begin to identify the most pressing areas of concern. With this information, you can use this book to start investigating and resolving these problems one at a time. In chapter 2, we talked about how these many obstacles are like straws on the camel's back. As the burden increases, you feel less and less able to manage diabetes, leading to diabetes burnout. This is the time to begin freeing yourself of this burden, lightening the load of your diabetes one "straw" at a time.

Each of the four major factors, or problem areas, is linked to a specific section of this book. Your response to part B on Worksheet 3.3 (indicating your highest score) can guide you to where to begin.

Overcoming Problems with Day-to-Day Self-Care

If your biggest problem area is the day-to-day struggle with self-care, you should begin with section II, "Diabetes Self-Care." You can read all of the chapters in this section or

WORKSHEET 3.2: WHAT'S DRIVING YOU CRAZY ABOUT DIABETES?

Directions: As on Worksheet 3.1, several potential problem areas that people with diabetes may experience are listed below. Consider the degree to which each of the items may have distressed or bothered you *during the past month* and circle the appropriate number. Remember that if you feel that a particular item is not a bother or problem, you will circle 1. If it is very bothersome, you will circle 6.

STRUGGLES WITH SELF-CARE:

	Not a problem		Moderate problem		Serious problem	
1. Feeling that I can't control my eating.	1	2	3	4	5	6
2. Feeling constantly deprived around food and eating.	1	2	3	4	5	6
3. Feeling that I am not sticking closely enough to a good meal plan.	1	2	3	4	5	6
4. Feeling that I am not getting enough physical exercise.	1	2	3	4	5	6
5. Feeling that I am not checking my blood sugars frequently enough.	1	2	3	4	5	6
6. Feeling that I am not taking the correct amount of insulin or pills often enough (taking less, or more, than I should).	1	2	3	4	5	6
7. Feeling unclear about exactly what or how much I should be doing to take care of my diabetes properly.	1	2	3	4	5	6
8. Not feeling knowledgeable enough about diabetes and diabetes self-care.	1	2	3	4	5	6

WORKSHEET 3.2: WHAT'S DRIVING YOU CRAZY ABOUT DIABETES? *(continued)*

YOUR SOCIAL RELATIONSHIPS:

	Not a problem		Moderate problem		Serious problem	
9. Feeling that there is no one in my life with whom I can talk openly about my feelings about diabetes.	1	2	3	4	5	6
10. Feeling that my friends or family treat me as if I were more fragile or sicker than I really am.	1	2	3	4	5	6
11. Feeling alone with diabetes.	1	2	3	4	5	6
12. Feeling that my friends or family act like "diabetes police" (nag me about eating properly, testing blood sugars, or not trying hard enough).	1	2	3	4	5	6
13. Feeling that my friends or family don't give me the support or help I need to take good care of my diabetes.	1	2	3	4	5	6
14. Feeling that my friends or family don't appreciate how difficult living with diabetes can be.	1	2	3	4	5	6
15. Feeling that I can't tell my doctor what is really on my mind.	1	2	3	4	5	6
16. Feeling that my doctor doesn't take my concerns seriously enough.	1	2	3	4	5	6

WORKSHEET 3.2: WHAT'S DRIVING YOU CRAZY ABOUT DIABETES? *(continued)*

YOUR ATTITUDES AND FEELINGS:

	Not a problem		Moderate problem		Serious problem	
17. Feeling depressed much of the time.	1	2	3	4	5	6
18. Feeling that I cannot "get going."	1	2	3	4	5	6
19. Feeling anxious much of the time.	1	2	3	4	5	6
20. Not feeling confident in my day-to-day ability to manage diabetes.	1	2	3	4	5	6
21. Feeling very frightened when I think about the possibility of long-term complications from diabetes.	1	2	3	4	5	6
22. Feeling that I will end up with serious long-term complications, no matter what I do.	1	2	3	4	5	6
23. Feeling that I must be perfect in my diabetes management.	1	2	3	4	5	6
24. Feeling angry, scared, and/or depressed when I think about living with diabetes.	1	2	3	4	5	6

let your responses to part C on Worksheet 3.3 (indicating your greatest areas of concern) guide you to the chapters you need:

▮ If your problems are centered on food, you might begin with chapter 4, "Ten Good Reasons Why It's Impossible to Follow a Healthy Meal Plan (and What to Do about Them)." If nighttime overeating

WORKSHEET 3.2: WHAT'S DRIVING YOU CRAZY ABOUT DIABETES? *(continued)*

YOUR STRESSES:

	Not a problem		Moderate problem		Serious problem	
25. Feeling that there is too much stress in my life.	1	2	3	4	5	6
26. Feeling that there are too many demands on my time.	1	2	3	4	5	6
27. Feeling that my life seems too boring.	1	2	3	4	5	6
28. Worrying about the financial burden of diabetes care.	1	2	3	4	5	6
29. Feeling that my blood sugars often swing wildly, no matter how hard I try.	1	2	3	4	5	6
30. Feeling frustrated that getting my blood sugars in better control has caused me to gain weight.	1	2	3	4	5	6
31. Worrying about low-blood-sugar reactions.	1	2	3	4	5	6
32. Not feeling the warning signs of low blood sugars like I used to.	1	2	3	4	5	6
	1	2	3	4	5	6

is your personal demon, consider chapter 5, "The Werewolf Syndrome."

∎ If your problems are focused on medication usage, you might begin with chapter 6, "Muddling by with Diabetes Medications."

∎ Are your biggest worries linked to blood glucose monitoring? Then consider starting with chapter 7, "Ten Good Reasons to Hate Blood Glucose Monitoring (and What to Do about Them)."

WORKSHEET 3.3: IDENTIFYING YOUR PROBLEM AREAS IN DIABETES

A. Of the four major areas on Worksheet 3.2, the following are problematic for me (record all areas where you scored greater than 16):

1. _____
2. _____
3. _____
4. _____

B. My biggest diabetes problem area seems to be (record your highest scoring area; if there is a tie, select the one that you believe is most important):

_____

C. Within that biggest problem area, I have the following special concerns (please record the 2 or 3 highest of your responses within this area; if there are more than 3, please select the ones you believe are most important):

1. _____
2. _____
3. _____

D. My second biggest diabetes problem area seems to be (record your second highest scoring area; if there is a tie, select the one you think is most important):

_____

E. Within that second biggest problem area, I have the following special concerns (please record the 2 or 3 highest of your responses within this area; if there are more than 3, please select the ones you believe are most important):

1. _____
2. _____
3. _____

F. My greatest area of strength seems to be (of any problem areas where you scored less than 16, consider whether any of those may represent a source of strength for you and then record here):

_____

NOTE: If none of your four scores on Worksheet 3.2 were greater than 16, you may still have specific areas of concern that were not easily identified through use of this method. Please examine your responses again and note any that were scored either 5 or 6. Record these in part C. Also, if only one of your scores was greater than 16, you will need to skip parts D and E.

- If your problems are focused on exercise, you might begin with chapter 8, "Ten Good Reasons to Avoid Exercise (and What to Do about Them)."
- Perhaps your concerns are broader, and you feel uncertain about "exactly what or how much I should be doing to take care of my diabetes properly." In that case, you should read all of section II and give special attention to chapter 9, "Harnessing Your Expectations: The Art of Developing Goals and Action Plans."
- If your problems result from a lack of knowledge about diabetes, you should make it a priority to enroll in your local hospital's diabetes education program or to call your local office of the American Diabetes Association to locate a good education program in your community. This is vitally important; there is no substitute for being informed!

Overcoming Problems Related to Feelings and Attitudes

If your biggest problem area involves your feelings and attitudes about diabetes, you should begin with section III, "Feelings and Attitudes." You can read all of the chapters in this section or let your responses to part C on Worksheet 3.3 guide you to the chapters you need:

- If you are anxious about the possibility of long-term complications, you might start with chapter 10, "Worrying about Long-Term Complications: The Uses and Misuses of Fear."
- If your problems involve depression, you might begin with chapter 11, "Depression and Diabetes: A Tough Combination."

- If your problems are focused on feeling angry, scared, or depressed about diabetes, chapter 11 and chapter 12, "What You Don't Know Can't Hurt You (or Can It?): Understanding and Overcoming Denial," might be good places to begin.

- If anxiety is a major concern, where you start will depend on the focus of your anxiety. If you are concerned that feelings of anxiety lead to overeating, then consider chapter 4. If you are anxious about hypoglycemia, you might start with chapter 17, "Worrying about Hypoglycemia."

- If you are not feeling confident that you can manage diabetes or if you are driving yourself crazy thinking that you must handle your diabetes perfectly, you might begin with chapter 12. Chapter 18, "When Good Actions Don't Lead to Good Results: The Blood Sugar Fairy and Other Uplifting Tales," should also be helpful.

Overcoming Problems with Social Relationships

If your biggest problem area involves your social relationships, you should begin with section IV, "Friends, Family, and Health Care Providers." Again you can read all of the chapters in this section or let your responses to part C guide you to the chapters you need:

- Feeling unsupported by your friends and family or feeling isolated with diabetes? Then consider starting with chapter 13, "The Secret of the Smoking Room."

- If your problems are focused on feeling blamed or hassled by your friends or family, you might begin with chapter 14, "The Diabetes Police."

■ If your problems are focused on feeling unsatisfied with your relationship with your doctor or other health care providers, you might begin with chapter 15, "Working with Your Health Care Team: The Agony and the Ecstasy."

Overcoming Environmental Stresses

If your biggest problem area concerns your environmental stresses, you should begin with section V, "Life Stresses/ Diabetes Stresses." You can read all of the chapters in the section or let your responses to part C on Worksheet 3.3 guide you to the chapters you need:

■ If your problems center on global feelings of being stressed or overwhelmed, you might begin with chapter 16, "How Stress Influences Diabetes (and What to Do about It)."
■ If your problems are focused on worries about hypoglycemia, you might start with chapter 17.
■ If you are discouraged because your efforts don't seem to be paying off (leading to disillusioning results like weight gain, more hypoglycemia, or erratic blood sugars that make no sense), you might begin with chapter 18. You should also consider reading the chapters in section II, "Diabetes Self-Care."

MEL'S FIRST STEPS TOWARD OVERCOMING BURNOUT

To illustrate how this exercise might be helpful, consider the case of Mel, whom you met in chapter 1. By completing the exercise, Mel learned some important things about himself. First, his diabetes burnout score from Worksheet

3.1 was 30, an extremely high score that confirmed for him how very overwhelmed he felt. Though he obviously knew he had been struggling with diabetes for many years, it was jarring to see this result and to realize how serious a problem this really was. It was as though the invisible had suddenly become visible, and Mel realized that he could no longer avoid addressing this terrible problem.

On Worksheet 3.2, his individual scores revealed that he was significantly distressed by all four major factors, which was not a big surprise given his high score from the first worksheet. However, Mel noticed that there were sizeable differences in his four scores. These differences were clarified when he completed Worksheet 3.3, which helped Mel to identify his greatest concerns about diabetes and to point the way toward overcoming burnout. As he studied the completed Worksheet 3.3, he realized that he needed to focus his initial efforts on changing his feelings about diabetes (especially his fear, anger, and sense of hopelessness about complications) as well as his self-care behaviors (confronting his discomfort with blood glucose monitoring, his dislike of meal planning, and his lack of current knowledge about diabetes care).

Toward these ends, he decided to begin with chapter 10 and chapter 12 to learn about dealing with fear and denial. He would then move on to chapters 4 and 6, concerning meal planning and blood glucose monitoring. In addition, he committed himself to enrolling in the diabetes education program at his local hospital. After years of inaction and burnout, Mel had succeeded in identifying the size and extent of his problem as well as his primary areas of diabetes-related concern, and he had put together an initial plan for action. It would be a bumpy but ultimately gratifying ride, for Mel was now well on the path toward making peace with diabetes.

Like Mel, you may now have a clearer sense of the scope of your battle with diabetes, the major areas of concern that need to be addressed, the strengths you bring to this task, and an initial plan for how to use this book to address those problems. If you have any confusion about how to proceed, read the remaining chapters in order. As you continue your journey through this book, you will pick up new ideas and strategies for overcoming the hassles of diabetes and will find opportunities to give structure to your planning. You will meet other people who have struggled with their diabetes, and you'll hear some sad stories and some funny ones. Keep an open mind and open heart, and let's keep going!

SECTION II
Diabetes Self-Care

CHAPTER 4
Ten Good Reasons Why It's Impossible to Follow a Healthy Meal Plan (and What to Do about Them)

This chapter is not about how to lose weight. It is not about meal planning, carbohydrate counting, or how to understand the food pyramid. There are no recipes. This chapter assumes you have an idea about *what* to eat and *how* to eat well, but that you are continuing to struggle anyway. Dietary knowledge is certainly important, but it is not enough for most people. Even if you know everything there is to know about the value of fruits and vegetables, the importance of fiber, and the balancing of carbohydrate intake throughout the day, the odds are good that you are still finding it difficult to follow a healthy meal plan. Consider the cases of Andrew and Katherine:

Andrew was a 45-year-old electrician who had been diagnosed with type 1 diabetes 24 years earlier. He had been on an intensive insulin regimen for many years and checked his blood glucose at least five times each day. Despite all this effort, his blood glucose level was typically around 220 mg/dl or higher. One of the main problems, as Andrew explained it to me, was food: "If I could just go without eating, everything would be fine. I hate food and love food, all at the same time." Andrew knew how to eat well and tried to follow a healthy meal plan, but his work schedule changed so often that he was lucky ever to find time for meals. And when it was time to eat, he would simply seek out whatever was convenient and tasty.

Unfortunately, this meant that Andrew was typically consuming few fruits and vegetables and very little fiber. At the same time, he was packing in a fair amount of junk food each day. He tried to pay attention to how the various foods affected his blood glucose and to match it with insulin, but this was never very successful. Feeling increasingly discouraged by his blood glucose results, Andrew began to check less and less often. Whenever he took the time to think about it, he felt like a failure and worried about the future of his health, but he just couldn't figure out what to do about it.

Katherine had battled with food—and with her weight—for many long years. At one time or another, she had tried almost every major diet program in America. In most of the programs, she was successful at first. But success never lasted. Eventually, she would tire of the various eating restrictions and would resume her old habits, such as snacking on chocolate chip cookies in the afternoon and eating high-fat, vegetable-free dinners. In each case, Katherine eventually regained all of her lost weight—and more.

By the time I met her, the battle with food was all but over. At 280 pounds, she had never been heavier. Now at age 54, she had developed heart disease and high blood pressure, and her type 2 diabetes was only being controlled with very large doses of insulin. Katherine longed to feel better, to be healthier, and to lose weight. But she felt hopeless that she could ever truly curb her cravings and follow a healthier meal plan.

EATING WELL AIN'T EASY

There are many people in situations similar to those of Katherine and Andrew. And this points to the fact that sticking to a healthy meal plan is probably the toughest aspect of diabetes care. Recent surveys have indicated that 10–24% of patients with diabetes rarely or never follow their health care team's dietary recommendations. Of course, this doesn't mean that the remaining 76–90% of patients are eating perfectly. Most people find it difficult to follow a healthy meal plan faithfully over long periods of time. After all, it's not easy to change lifelong habits. For example, although most people with diabetes seem to improve their eating habits after learning about the importance of healthy eating, these gains are often only temporary.

WHAT'S SO TOUGH ABOUT EATING WELL?

Why is following a healthy meal plan such a struggle? After all, there is powerful and convincing research evidence that—just like your mother always told you—a diet that is low in saturated fat, high in fiber, and loaded with fruits and vegetables can

- significantly lower your risk for heart disease and cancer
- provide you with more energy every day
- help you to manage your weight
- have a beneficial effect on your diabetes management (especially if you are balancing carbohydrates throughout the day)

Sounds good, doesn't it? Knowing about all these remarkable benefits may inspire you to *want* to follow a healthy meal plan. It may even get you started on the right path. But, as it did for Katherine and Andrew, life often gets in the way.

If you have tried unsuccessfully to follow a healthy meal plan, it is not because you are stupid or lack will-power. Although you recognize the benefits of healthy eating, you may still be overwhelmed by the many personal, social, and environmental barriers that block you from following such a meal plan. And, in fact, there are some good reasons why following a healthy meal plan seems all but impossible. Take a look at the top 10:

1. You are not exactly certain *how* to follow a healthy meal plan. Perhaps you know about the value of fruits and vegetables and the importance of dietary fiber. That does-n't necessarily mean that you understand how to put that knowledge to use in your daily life. What exactly does it mean to "follow a healthy meal plan"? *The primary reason why most people find it too difficult to follow a healthy meal plan is that they don't really have a plan at all.* If you just have a vague sense that you should somehow be "eating better," that's going to be a difficult plan to follow!

Unfortunately, even after a long meeting with your doctor or dietitian, you may still be unsure about exactly how you should be eating. Perhaps your health care provider gave you recommendations that were too imprecise (for example, "You need to cut out some of the fat in your diet"). Perhaps he or she overwhelmed you with so many dietary recommendations that you don't even know where to start. Or perhaps you were having a hard time listening. Without a doubt, it is impossible to follow a healthy meal plan if you do not have a clear idea of exactly what you should be doing.

2. Your vision of a healthy meal plan is unrealistic. Many people are convinced that there are only two ways of eating. Both ways are rather extreme: the *right and virtuous* approach versus your *normal* way of eating. The right and virtuous approach means a life of restrictions. As one of my patients, Fred, described it, "My doctor told me about the importance of a healthy meal plan, which— as best as I can tell—means I'm only allowed to eat bird-seed all day." The right and virtuous approach means a life without chocolate, chips, pizza, or anything else that you might find tasty. It means eating perfectly every day. The right and virtuous approach means never, ever cheating. In contrast, your normal way of eating probably means a vacation from being right and virtuous. It means freedom: being able to eat anything you want, whenever you want.

When you become convinced that you must follow the right and virtuous approach, all of life can then be divided into two different time zones: those times when you are on the right and virtuous diet and those times when you are off. And once you develop this split in your mind, you have set yourself up for feeling like a failure. When you cannot be perfect—and no one can—it is easy to become discouraged. Once you realize that you cannot adopt the right and virtuous approach as a practical, long-term way of living, it is likely that you will eventually admit defeat and return to your old, "imperfect" way of eating.

3. There are too many temptations everywhere, and it is too hard to resist them. Perhaps you are trying to avoid ice cream, but there is a quart in the freezer (for the kids, of course) and it's calling your name. Maybe you have been doing your best to stop snacking between meals, but you just saw a pizza commercial on TV and, boy, it sure looked good. There is no doubt about it, we are surrounded by temptations to eat foods that are high in fat, high in sugar, and low in nutritional value—on billboards, on TV, at the movie theater, in the neighborhood, at your neighbor's, and even in your own home. In a fast-food culture like America, it is so easy to give into those temptations. Who could possibly resist?

4. Life is too stressful. After a tough day, you may automatically want to reward yourself with a favorite "comfort food." If you have had a difficult interaction with someone or you are feeling particularly angry, sad, anxious, or lonely, you may seek out a favorite food to soothe or calm yourself. Unfortunately, almost no one tends to find comfort in carrot sticks! The more common culprits are potato chips, cookies, chocolate, and ice cream—and usually not in small amounts. The consumption of comfort foods is a popular strategy for reducing stress. Unfortunately, it doesn't work very well! Stresses and worries may vanish for a time, but they soon return. In fact, after straying seriously from your meal plan, you may even feel worse about yourself and become more stressed.

5. Eating at restaurants or at social events is just too hard. Perhaps you would like to reduce the fat in your diet, but your favorite Italian restaurant always brings that wonderful garlic bread to your table. And it's just dripping with butter. How can you possibly resist? Indeed, few restaurants in America support a nutritious approach to eating. Generally speaking, what is advertised and sold in this nation is tasty, high-fat dishes in very large portions. It is difficult to go into most restaurants and find a healthy choice. To be successful, you often need to grill your waitress or waiter about how different entrees are prepared—"What exactly is in that clam dip?" But this requires a degree of assertiveness that is often exhausting, may be irritating to others, and may draw unwanted attention to you.

6. It takes too much time and effort. For those people whose days are already busy enough, it may seem hard to find the time to follow a healthy meal plan. The typical American approach to eating is based on convenience. And convenience foods—TV dinners, take-out pizza, macaroni and cheese, donuts, and burgers from your favorite fast-food joint—are rarely healthy choices. Buying and preparing fresh vegetables, searching out recipes for healthier meals, or seeking out more wholesome alternatives for late afternoon snacking may all sound like good ideas, but how could you possibly find the extra time each day to make any of these things happen? Worse yet, it takes a conscious effort to break old eating habits. You know it would be smart to make the effort, but it is so much easier to just keep doing what you are doing. This is especially true when you also have to worry about pleasing the other people in your household, who have their own established tastes and desires.

7. Every time you've tried to follow a healthy meal plan, the results have been discouraging. Could anything sap your motivation more than this? If past attempts to follow a healthy meal plan haven't led to positive results, no wonder you don't feel excited to try again! One of my patients, Reggie, explained it this way: "It happens over and over. Yesterday, for example, I followed my prescribed meal plan almost perfectly, and I even skipped dinner. So I woke up this morning and my blood sugar was 300 mg/dl! This is just ridiculous. Why should I bother even trying?" And then there was Muriel, who was in tears at our very first meeting: "When my doctor told me I had diabetes and that I needed to start taking pills to control it, I knew it was finally time to lose some weight. To achieve this, the dietitian helped me to set up a good meal plan, which I have now been faithfully following for several weeks. I thought I was doing great, until I arrived here at the clinic this morning and found that I had not even lost a pound! I feel so defeated that I just want to give up."

Like Reggie and Muriel, you may find that it's easier to stick with tough changes in your eating when you are getting positive feedback, such as favorable changes in blood glucose, cholesterol levels, or other important markers of health. When you don't get this feedback, it can seem like your efforts don't really matter, which can be terribly hard on your morale.

8. You get no cooperation or support from your family. When you are living in a household of vegetable-hating, cookie-crazed savages, it may be quite challenging to follow a healthy meal plan. The lucky people are those who have spouses, families, or close friends who are rooting for their success and are also willing to join them in a healthier approach to eating. When your loved ones are choosing to eat as you do, you are unlikely to feel as deprived or as swayed by temptation. However, if your loved ones don't know about your diabetes needs or seem to ignore or downplay your desire to adopt a healthy meal plan, trouble is likely. For example, your spouse may say, "You go ahead and change how you are eating in any way that you want, but that doesn't mean that the rest of us have to suffer or be deprived." Attitudes like these are a recipe for disaster. It is difficult enough to make long-term healthy changes in eating, but when you must make them without any support from friends or family (or, worse yet, in the face of your loved ones' refusal to support you), it can become almost impossible.

9. Eating healthfully is boring. It is a widely believed folktale that adopting a healthy approach toward eating means living an empty, rigid, and painful life, one that is devoid of all pleasure but loaded with carrot and celery sticks. And there is some truth to this: Without some effort and planning, following a healthy meal plan can easily become boring. This is especially likely when you adopt a meal plan that is too strict ("I can only eat these particular foods at these particular times"). A meal plan this strict can take the flexibility and enjoyment out of eating. Food can begin to seem like simple fuel or, worse yet, a medication. Boredom is also likely to set in when you are focusing on the pain of what you *shouldn't* be eating ("I really must eat fewer candy bars"), rather than the pleasure of what you *could* be eating ("I am looking forward to having more fresh fruit in my diet").

Finally, there is the problem of dietary fat. Because of our biology, we are delighted by foods that are high in artery-clogging fat—think of ice cream, donuts, and potato chips. Worse yet, one of the primary ways in which we Americans make food tasty is to add fat, lots of it— think of fried foods, double-cheese pizza, or bagels slathered with cream cheese. Because a healthier approach to eating includes—at least for most people— lowering the amount of fat in your diet, meals and snacks could begin to seem pretty bland if you don't find other ways to make food more flavorful. Indeed, this may be the primary reason why following a healthy meal plan eventually becomes too difficult. People begin to feel bored and deprived. And it is easy to lose the desire to eat well when it starts to feel like a punishment.

10. It is hard to say no. When offered a tasty but unhealthy snack at a social gathering, at a friend's home, or even at your own dinner table, it can be awfully tough to turn it down. When Aunt Betsy begs you to try a piece of her chocolate cream pie (which she made just for you), when your friends order the bacon and cheese potato skins as an appetizer and expect you to share it with them, or when your neighbor invites you over for a big bowl of ice cream, it is so much more convenient, easy, and pleasurable to say yes. After all, it would be impolite to do otherwise! And who wishes to make a big fuss at times like these? Given the social circumstances, you probably want to fit in with everyone else. You might feel that the last thing you want to do is to draw attention to your diabetes. So it seems better just to keep quiet and start eating. If this is truly a rare occurrence, there is probably little reason to worry. But it can become very difficult to follow a healthy meal plan when this is happening day after day or when an event like this serves to open your own personal floodgates: "Since I've blown it now with Aunt Betsy's pie, I might as well just keep eating for the rest of the day."

OVERCOMING THE BARRIERS TO HEALTHY EATING

As you consider the barriers to eating well, you may be growing more and more discouraged. But wait a minute! Following a healthy meal plan is not impossible, and it doesn't have to be painful. So consider which of the 10 reasons, or barriers, may apply to you, and let's review the seven major strategies for getting past them. By using these strategies, you may discover a sense of accomplishment and take pleasure in eating well.

1. With your health care team, develop a meal plan that is clear and reasonable for you—especially if you're not sure *how* to follow a meal plan (reason 1) or your meal plan is unrealistic (reason 2). If you began following a healthy meal plan tomorrow morning, what exactly would you do? What would you have for breakfast? Or lunch? Would you need to shop this evening for some new food products? If you are not certain, get some help. Set up an appointment with a diabetes-knowledgeable dietitian or one of your other health care providers.

While it is true that you want to challenge yourself to follow as healthy a meal plan as possible, it is equally important that you be kind to yourself. You should start

---

SEVEN STRATEGIES FOR OVERCOMING THE BARRIERS TO FOLLOWING A HEALTHY MEAL PLAN

1. With your health care team, develop a meal plan that is clear and reasonable for you.
2. Modify your eating environments to support your efforts.
3. In the face of meal planning disappointments, get perspective.
4. Make use of the principles of "structured cheating."
5. Focus your attention on the new habits you are planning to start, not the old habits you are trying to stop.
6. If your daily life seems boring, take action.
7. In challenging social situations, make use of assertiveness strategies.

---

with a meal plan change that can realistically be accomplished. Think of it this way: if you have been consuming a high-fat diet every day for the past few decades, is it reasonable to think that you can suddenly give up most of your favorite high-fat foods *forever* and switch to a low-fat diet beginning tomorrow? Probably not.

So don't set yourself up with unrealistic expectations. While it is important to have ambitious and specific long-range goals, such as reducing your daily fat intake from 40% of your daily diet to 20%, you must begin with a reasonable short-range plan that moves you in the general direction of your long-range goals. For example, "At dinnertime over the next week, I will add at least a cup of vegetables and cut back on the amount of red meat I consume." Following this practical approach to change, you are more likely to meet your goals, which can help you feel a real sense of accomplishment. Feeling more confident, you will be more willing to make and maintain further eating changes. You will inch your way ever closer to a truly healthy meal plan.

2. Modify your eating environments to support your efforts—especially if you feel it's too hard to resist temptation (reason 3), it's difficult to eat healthfully at restaurants or social events (reason 5), or eating well takes too much time and effort (reason 6). This is common sense. You can plan ahead and rearrange your kitchen, your daily driving routes, or even your restaurant choices to make healthy eating more convenient and make unhealthy eating inconvenient. Try the following:

- Refuse to purchase your most tempting snacks.
- Rearrange your schedule so that you are busy during your most vulnerable, snack-prone moments. For

instance, plan a walk during the afternoon when you are most likely to binge on potato chips.

■ Put the least healthy foods on the highest or most distant shelf in the kitchen.

■ Find an alternative route to your destination that doesn't take you past your favorite fast-food restaurant. If you can't drive by the donut shop without stopping in for a dozen, take a different street.

■ Seek out new restaurants where healthy choices are available.

■ In restaurants, consider asking your server to help your efforts by not bringing garlic bread, chips, or other less healthy sides to your table.

■ Make changes in how you shop or cook that make it less time-consuming to follow a healthy meal plan. For example, buy vegetables that have already been washed and presliced, involve your family members in helping to prepare healthy meals, or investigate new lines of frozen entrees that are both more nutritious and tasty.

A dietitian who is knowledgeable about diabetes is likely to be a terrific source of creative ideas for developing a healthy *and practical* meal plan that is not overwhelming in terms of time or effort. Remember that the underlying idea in all of these suggestions is straightforward: take action and be creative about making simple changes in your environment, no matter where you are, to support your efforts. For more ideas, see chapter 5.

3. In the face of meal planning disappointments, get perspective—especially if you've had discouraging results in the past (reason 7) or think healthy eating is boring (reason 9). If it seems that your best efforts to follow a healthy meal plan only lead to discouraging results, your first step should be to make time for a reality check. Why? Because your results may not be as discouraging as you think. Take Reggie, for example. Even if he carefully follows his meal plan every day, there will be times when his blood glucose level is going to do something wacky— soaring higher or dropping for no obvious reason. Even a carefully followed meal plan will occasionally result in unusual blood glucose responses.

To avoid becoming discouraged, the most important thing to do is to adopt a broader perspective. Following a good meal plan may have led to frustrating results yesterday morning, but does it have to ruin today? Although it may be hard to remember, perhaps your efforts have been beneficial to your blood glucose levels on most mornings in the past (as well as afternoons and evenings). Pay attention to the *pattern* of your blood glucose over a number of days. Just as importantly, be sure to have a glycated hemoglobin (HbA1c) test completed on a regular basis. Let this be one of your main guides to evaluating your own progress.

Although it required a good deal of patience, this approach turned out to be quite helpful for Reggie. Rather than letting each and every blood glucose result sway his feelings, Reggie arranged to have an HbA1c test completed every 3 months. After carefully following his new meal plan for 9 months, these tests clearly showed that Reggie's average blood glucose levels were steadily dropping. This was tremendously reassuring. It helped Reggie realize that his efforts really were paying off.

If you are trying to lose weight, it is even more important that you maintain a broader perspective and stick to reasonable expectations. Even with the most restrictive of diets, real weight loss can be painfully slow. And if, like Muriel, you have simultaneously begun to improve your blood glucose control, weight loss may be even slower. A significant drop in blood glucose level means that your body is now absorbing calories more effectively from the foods you eat. Thus, it is common for people who are beginning a new diabetes medication (especially if it is insulin or of the class of oral medications known as sulfonylureas) to *gain* weight, at least initially. You can see how this information could have really helped Muriel. The fact that her weight stayed the same over the first few weeks was actually quite an achievement. Following a healthier meal plan, with a special emphasis on weight loss, had actually been successful. With this information and more realistic expectations for the future pace of her weight loss, Muriel felt heartened, rather than discouraged, by these results.

4. Make use of the principles of "structured cheating" (this should be valuable if any of the reasons apply to you). If you have a meal plan that is too strict or too boring for you or one that makes you feel too deprived, you won't keep following it. For example, perhaps you believe that you must live without chocolate donuts for the rest of your life, but—so far—you haven't been able to go even a few days without one. So let's be honest about this and consider your actual track record so far. Is it reasonable to believe that you will be able to follow your current meal plan faithfully forever? That you will never "cheat"? In fact, by struggling to restrict your eating in a way that is truly impractical for you at this time, you may be guaranteeing that you will continue to salivate about donuts every day.

So what is the answer to this problem? To mentally flog yourself ever harder, hoping against hope that you will suddenly develop perfect willpower? Probably not. The best solution may be to compromise. At this time in your life, if you can't live in a world without chocolate donuts (or pizza, or hot fudge sundaes, or whatever), then don't! After all, it's not really *cheating* (which is a terribly silly term), it's just *eating*. Working together with your health care team, make sure to include donuts in your life, but do it in a way that minimizes any harm. Think of this approach, often the first step toward a healthier meal plan, as *structured cheating*.

How do you compromise on something like eating donuts? Well, you will need to use a little common sense. In reality, continuing to consume a dozen chocolate donuts every day is probably not a good idea, especially if you are trying to manage your blood glucose and weight. On the other hand, a few donuts each week may not be such a bad thing at all. And by planning ahead for eating a donut, you may able to reduce the impact of those donuts on your blood glucose (by adjusting your medications, exercise, or other food intake, for example). Most importantly, by deliberately including some of your favorite foods in your weekly meal plan—no matter how fattening or "bad" they are—you will weaken their ability to tempt you throughout the week. You will probably end up eating fewer donuts, and you will feel more in control of your eating. By following this approach, you won't be eating *perfectly*, but you are likely to be much more successful in following a reasonably healthy meal plan.

5. Focus your attention on the new habits you are planning to start, not the old habits you are trying to

stop—especially if you feel it's too hard to resist temptation (reason 3), it's too difficult to eat healthfully at restaurants or social events (reason 5), or eating healthfully is boring (reason 9). Like Katherine, you may be driving yourself crazy trying to cut down on your afternoon snacking or your frequent trips to fast-food restaurants. Unfortunately, trying to deprive yourself just doesn't seem to work very well. In fact, this probably makes you desire those "forbidden foods" even more strongly. As long as you stay focused on the many foods that you are trying to cut back on, continuously thinking about what you are missing, you are likely to be doomed. Instead, pay attention to the new foods or new actions that you are trying to bring in to your life. With some planning, you should find that these new, positive changes will automatically begin to interfere with your old, unhealthy eating habits.

Katherine found this to be a useful approach. In place of battling with herself about the amount of meat and other high-fat foods she was consuming at dinner, she decided to concentrate her attention on eating a large helping of vegetables each evening. Rather than continuing to torture herself uselessly about her afternoon snacking (on large numbers of chocolate chip cookies), she focused her thoughts on what she would begin to add to her afternoons: a brisk walk through the neighborhood. This change in thinking really helped. Instead of feeling passive, helpless, and deprived, she felt energized by the realization that her new, positive actions could really make a difference: By consuming a higher volume of vegetables at dinner, she became too full to finish her typically high-fat dinners. And by walking each afternoon, she began to lose interest in snacking.

6. If your daily life seems boring, take action—especially if you feel it's too hard to resist temptation (reason 3), life is too stressful (reason 4), or healthy eating is too boring (reason 9). For some people, eating is—unfortunately—the only enjoyable, stimulating aspect of their daily lives. When the majority of your evenings, for example, are spent alone and consist of little more than watching a series of dull television shows, it is no wonder that the prospect of consuming an enormous hot fudge sundae each night may fill you with unstoppable glee. So if you have not succeeded in following a healthy meal plan, the problem may have nothing to do with your attitudes toward food. Consider the broader possibility that you may be suffering from a lack of excitement, challenge, or stimulation in your life. By taking action to address these areas of boredom, you may find that your need to seek solace in pastries or desserts may weaken considerably.

Consider the case of Peter, for example. Since retiring several years earlier, he had found it more and more difficult to manage his own eating. Despite his best efforts, he would typically snack throughout the day, usually on sweets and other junk food. Not surprisingly, his blood glucose levels had begun to rise and it was likely that he would need to start insulin soon. As it turned out, there was an easier solution. A bright and lively man, Peter was clearly bored and irritated by retirement. He missed the intellectual challenge of his work as well as the companionship of his fellow employees. As a consequence of our conversations, he realized how bored he really was and decided to take action: volunteering his time at a local museum. Within several weeks, his whole attitude toward snacking began to change. Now that he was finding his life more stimulating every day, he no longer needed to seek out junk food snacks to relieve his boredom. And as his eating improved, his blood glucose soon stabilized and began to drop.

Give some thought to the degree of boredom in your own life. If you are feeling understimulated, lonely, or unchallenged, consider making a change. Even a small change could make a big difference. Volunteering your time (as Peter did), developing a hobby, making a new friend, turning off the television, or joining a new group or organization—anything that will help you to feel more engaged and interested in the world—may reduce your cravings for food.

7. In challenging social situations, make use of assertiveness strategies—especially if you have a hard time saying no (reason 10). Having trouble turning down delicious foods when they are offered to you? One of the major reasons you may be uncomfortable saying no, especially when being offered food, is that you do not wish to convey a bad image of yourself. You don't want to be seen as rude, different, or sick ("Of course he can't eat foods like that, he has that terrible disease—diabetes"). Also, you probably don't want to offend the one who is offering. Being assertive means having and using your ability to say no, confidently and politely, while also putting forward a positive image of yourself. Whether you do or do not want to talk about your diabetes, this doesn't have to be difficult. Here are some tips that can help:

▌ Use "I" statements. For example, consider the differ-
ence between "Thanks, I don't want any potato skins right now" versus "Thanks, but potato skins really aren't good for me." By beginning your sentences

with "I," you are taking responsibility for your thoughts and feelings.

▌ When appropriate, acknowledge that you don't want to be rude. For instance, if your neighbor invites you for ice cream, don't be shy about stating all the different parts of your feelings. You might say, "Thanks for the offer, but I don't eat ice cream. I hope I haven't offended you. We should get together anyway." By communicating both parts of your message out loud (no ice cream for me *and* I don't want to hurt your feelings), you can feel more comfortable and confident about saying what you really mean.

▌ Recommend a more suitable, substitute action. If you would like to avoid the slice of homemade pie that Aunt Betsy is offering, try, "Thanks, it sure looks terrific, but not right now. Instead, I'd sure appreciate another slice of that delicious fruit." In this manner, you are taking control of the interaction, subtly shifting the conversation in a new, more healthy direction—away from further discussion of Aunt Betsy's pie and toward a more appropriate food choice.

AWARENESS AND ACTION

If you have diabetes, there is probably no greater frustration than the struggles around food. The good news is that it doesn't have to be this way. The keys to success are awareness and action. By paying careful attention to the barriers that block your path and by taking action to overcome those obstacles, you can change your whole way of thinking about food. You have seen how Katherine and others have used this approach to overcome the barriers that stood in their way. In fact, most of the people whom

BEYOND MEAL PLANNING STRUGGLES: EATING DISORDERS AND DIABETES

Day-to-day battles with eating and weight are tough enough, but things can become much worse when an eating disorder develops. If you have an eating disorder, you are probably feeling at war with food and with your body. You may feel ashamed, frustrated, isolated, depressed, and desperately out of control of your life. Tragically, eating disorders are common in America. As many as 8 million people are suffering right now. Although they can strike anyone, male or female, at almost any age, young women are at greatest risk. And research suggests that young women with type 1 diabetes are more likely to develop an eating disorder than young women without diabetes. In fact, among adolescent and young-adult women with type 1 diabetes, it appears that more than 1 in 10 are suffering with a diagnosable eating disorder.

There are three different types of eating disorders:

I *anorexia nervosa*, characterized by severely distorted body image, intense fear of weight gain, and extremely restricted eating

I *bulimia nervosa*, characterized by preoccupation with weight and fear of weight gain, and binge eating (consuming huge amounts of food in a short period of time) followed by purging—for example, by vomiting, by using laxatives, or in people with diabetes, by withholding insulin (see chapter 6)

I *binge eating disorder* (not yet a formal diagnosis, but perhaps the most common), characterized by preoccupation with weight and frequent binge eating, without the purging seen in bulimia

For someone with diabetes, any of these eating disorders is likely to mean big trouble. They are emotionally and physically exhausting, and—even more importantly—the medical consequences are likely to be severe. Among people with eating disorders (especially among people who are omitting insulin), glycated hemoglobin levels tend to be much higher and long-term complications develop much more rapidly. *(continued)*

BEYOND MEAL PLANNING STRUGGLES: EATING DISORDERS AND DIABETES (continued)

Eating Disorders Can Be Overcome!

You can beat even the most serious of eating disorders. But if you suspect that you are in the grips of one, you must seek professional help. It is extremely difficult to overcome an eating disorder on your own. You need someone to help you find the strength and skills to break such deadly habits and to help you feel good about yourself again. If you have been keeping your problem secret, it will be difficult to make that first call. The shame and guilt can be overwhelming. But you *can* do it.

You might start by confiding in a friend, a family member, or your doctor, but it is important to find a therapist—a psychiatrist, a psychologist, or a social worker—whom you trust and respect and who respects you. Most importantly, it should be someone who is skilled in the treatment of eating disorders as well as knowledgeable about diabetes. She or he will need to work closely with you and your diabetes care provider. Please, make the call right now!

you have met in this chapter are now following a healthy meal plan with greater success than ever before.

Remember Andrew from the beginning of this chapter? After some reflection, he realized that he had unrealistic expectations that were blocking his path. While he scolded himself for not eating perfectly, he finally recognized that a more reasonable plan of action, a compromise, was necessary. He didn't *want* to take the time away from his busy work schedule to worry about food, but he realized that he certainly *could* do so. At least, a little bit of time. After all, as an independent electrician, he was setting his own schedule. So he arranged each morning's schedule to allow himself 30 extra minutes to prepare and pack a healthy lunch and several nutritious snacks. Rather than grabbing a greasy cheeseburger and fries for lunch and pastries or candy bars for snacks, he began to eat tasty, low-fat sandwiches, fresh fruits, and fresh vegetable snacks. Not only did he enjoy his meals more, but he also found that he could more successfully adjust his insulin to match his intake. Tentatively at first, he began to check his blood glucose again throughout the day, and he was delighted by the results. His blood glucose levels were soon averaging 150 mg/dl, an impressive drop of 70 points.

By taking the time to identify your barriers and to try out even one of the seven strategies for overcoming them, you will be taking an important step toward making peace with food. You will start to bring a healthier and more satisfying way of eating into your life.

CHAPTER 5
The Werewolf Syndrome

Veronica was a 46-year-old woman with a flourishing career in the banking industry. Living with type 2 diabetes for the past 4 years, she had been trying to follow her doctor's recommendations, but was feeling aggravated with herself. She exercised regularly, checked her blood glucose several times each day, and ate three small, nutritious meals daily. In spite of all this, she was unable to get "good numbers." In fact, it had been many months since she had last seen a blood glucose reading under 220 mg/dl. Given these results, her doctor had told her that she would soon need to begin insulin.

Veronica knew that her problem was the evening hours. On a typical night, shortly after dinner, she would start to feel tense and uncomfortable. Seemingly against her will, she would skulk into the kitchen, nibbling quickly at whatever little goodies she could find (usually pie, cake, and cookies). She would then get angry with herself and retreat back to the family room. Throughout the evening, she would return to the kitchen again and again, devouring ever larger and larger amounts. And once this began, she found herself unable to stop. By the end of the evening, she was furious with herself and furious at diabetes. Even worse, as delicious as she imagined all her goodies would taste, she didn't really find them that satisfying anymore.

By the next morning, Veronica would have committed herself to redoubling her willpower and never letting another such evening occur, but—as the next evening approached—she knew she was all but powerless. In desperation, she had recently visited a dietitian who had helped her with new meal planning strategies, but this was to no avail. If anything, her nighttime overeating episodes were occurring more and more frequently.

In diabetes, there is no bigger battlefield and no greater frustration than food. On that battlefield, many different types of struggles may develop. And Veronica's battle with food, termed "the werewolf syndrome," is one of the most common problems. The term may not seem familiar to you, but most people actually know quite a bit about this type of struggle. Victims of the werewolf syndrome are those people who manage to follow a relatively healthy and well-balanced diet, *but only as long as the sun is up.* For as the moon rises, hair may begin to sprout on their faces, their eyes grow large, and their thoughts turn crazily to food, food, and more food. Soon they are on the prowl, and God help any goodies that they may come across!

Of course, the werewolf syndrome refers to the very common problem of nighttime overeating, which—in its more severe forms—can lead to overwhelming feelings of anxiety, aggravation, and guilt. And when you also have diabetes, you can see how werewolf eating could lead to some very serious problems.

No research study has yet documented how widespread the werewolf syndrome really is, but it is probably safe to assume that there are a lot of werewolves out there. When I have lectured about the werewolf syndrome to diabetes groups across the nation over the past several years, I have always noticed that the majority of each audience is nodding in understanding (and, often, with some slight embarrassment). Also, in our recent diabetes survey studies, my colleagues and I found that well over half of all patients reported at least some problem with controlling their eating. The odds are good that many, if not most, of those problems are occurring at night.

How can you identify the werewolf? As in Veronica's case, there are three common characteristics that all victims share:

■ They tend to eat fairly well during the daylight hours. However, they often make the mistake of eating "too well." They spend so much effort on limiting their daytime eating that their meals are often tiny, unsatisfying, or boring.

■ During the evening hours, they tend to lose control, often consuming large amounts of food, especially those "forbidden" foods that are certain to drive up blood glucose levels. Even though they may not be hungry at all, they feel powerless to stop these binges.

■ They tend to torment themselves. Rather than enjoying what they are eating, they end up feeling terribly depressed and guilty. Indeed, like the old tales of werewolves, they rarely take pleasure from their nightly forays. Because of these feelings, they will tend to feast alone. Unfortunately, no matter how much they punish themselves and no matter how strong their self-discipline may be, they are usually unable to prevent further bouts of werewolf eating.

As if living with diabetes isn't difficult enough all by itself! When you now introduce a werewolf into the house, you can be assured that diabetes will become even more difficult to manage. Why? Because frequent night-time eating is likely to lead to significant weight gain as well as chronically elevated blood glucose levels. It is therefore imperative to take action to understand and resolve this problem. If you are a victim of the werewolf syndrome, have courage. As you will soon see, the werewolf can be tamed.

HOW THE WEREWOLF IS UNLEASHED

The emergence of the mythical werewolf was usually linked to magical spells, the bite of another werewolf, or the rising of the full moon. Could these phenomena explain werewolf eating? Unfortunately, no. The real triggers are somewhat more mundane:

- stomach hunger
- eyeball hunger
- evening boredom
- unconscious eating
- difficult emotions

Stomach Hunger

Limited food intake during the daylight hours can lead to *stomach hunger*. If daytime meals are small, you may become quite hungry by the time evening rolls around. Maybe you have been dieting and are trying to eat as little as possible, maybe you are feeling so guilty about *last* night's appearance of the werewolf that you've decided to punish yourself by eating only carrot sticks today, or maybe you are trying to follow a diabetes meal plan that is just too limited and restricting for you. In any of these cases, your stomach growls at you louder and louder as the day progresses. By nighttime, despite all of your attempts at self-discipline, the urge to eat can no longer be resisted! Worse yet, when in a state of over-whelming hunger, you cannot be satisfied by small amounts of food. Instead, the mind and body overreact, becoming rav-enous. You eat and eat until you are stuffed. So werewolf eating can actually be triggered by attempts at dieting or other major food restrictions.

Eyeball Hunger

Unsatisfying food intake during the daylight hours can lead to *eyeball hunger*. Even though you may be eating plenty of food during the day, you may still find yourself hungry during the evening. While your stomach may be satisfied, your eyeballs, mouth, and brain may still feel famished. This can happen when you're feeling unsatisfied with your food choices throughout the day.

For example, Veronica's food intake during the day was more than sufficient to ward off stomach hunger during the evening, and yet she ate and ate during the night hours. However, Veronica's meals were totally uninteresting to her. As a card-carrying perfectionist, she had zealously followed the food choices that had been selected for her by the dietitian (designed to ensure that carbohydrates were balanced during the day, to avoid weight gain, and to provide good nutrition), without taking into account the importance of her own personal tastes and desires.

In other words, she was treating her meals as if they were merely fuel for her body's machine. Nothing that she ate was particularly enjoyable; as she described the situation, it seemed as if she was eating "nothing but rabbit food" all day. Thus, during the calm and quiet hours of the evening, with nothing else to distract her, a part of her brain would begin to revolt, seeking relief from this feeling of deprivation, and the prowl for truly satisfying foodstuffs (all the things she would not normally allow herself to have—like pie, cake, and cookies) would begin.

Consider how restrictive your own daytime eating may be. If your meal plan is too limiting (in terms of food *types*, not just food *amounts*), you may be depriving yourself of the joy of eating and the sense of satisfaction that your mind and body crave.

Evening Boredom

Feeling bored, dissatisfied, or lonely at night is a common trigger for werewolf eating. Perhaps you are watching television but aren't really interested in what is on. Perhaps you wish you had someone to talk to or to do something with, but there is no one at hand. At times like this, even though you are not hungry at all, a journey to the kitchen may serve as the only pleasure or stimulation that seems available. And this is understandable. Unfortunately, while boredom can lead to werewolf eating, most people discover that its not a very successful coping strategy. In other words, overeating doesn't do a very good job of relieving boredom.

Unconscious Eating

One of my patients described how she would innocently sit down to watch television each evening with a big box of cookies by her side. She would promise herself that she would only eat one or two, but then she would become engrossed in television. The next thing she knew, the box of cookies was "suddenly" empty, and there were crumbs all over her blouse. When this first happened, she was shocked. What had happened? Had someone broken into the house, knocked her unconscious, eaten all the cookies, and then spread crumbs all over her? As this continued night after night, it didn't take her long to realize that she wasn't dealing with a house thief. She was faced with something even worse—a werewolf!

Nighttime overeating may occur whenever you are preoccupied with some nonfood activity that is now linked, by habit, to eating. This can include reading, doing household chores, or watching television. One werewolf victim, for example, described how he automatically and unconsciously ate a large bag of Doritos each night as he read the newspaper. This was such a powerful and automatic behavior for him, one that he had done daily for so many years, that he completely ignored all the subtle but important body cues that might have helped him to cope more successfully. Remarkably, when he finally began to pay closer attention to his actions, he realized that he really wasn't that hungry and that he didn't really like the taste of Doritos anymore!

Difficult Emotions

If you're experiencing a difficult emotion like anger, sadness, anxiety, frustration, or loneliness, you may automatically seek to comfort yourself through eating. Veronica, for example, never knew why she felt so anxious each evening, but reaching out for her favorite foods was a comfortable and easy way to soothe herself. This is familiar to most of us. Eating—especially when it involves our favorite "comfort foods"—is a widely used strategy for emotional calming, in adults as well as children. Unfortunately, it is not a very effective strategy for managing stress. Regardless of how much you eat, the bad feelings don't recede for very long. Even worse, after a serious bout of werewolf eating, there is even more to feel bad about!

In addition, once a werewolf frenzy has begun, it is almost impossible to stop. Indeed, it is not uncommon to think, "Well, I've blown it now, so I might as well just keep eating, and I'll start afresh tomorrow." Now that permission is granted, the werewolf is fully unchained. The floodgates for eating are now spread wide! The next morning, to compensate for overeating the night before, the werewolf victim may start the new day by restricting his or her eating even more thoroughly. This is likely to lead to more hunger and even stronger feelings of deprivation, resulting in the return of the werewolf that very evening. Thus, the tragedy of this way of thinking, known as the diet-binge mentality, is that it all but ensures that the werewolf will be back night after night.

TAMING THE WEREWOLF

So what to do about the werewolf? Obviously, something greater than mere willpower is needed. For instance, consider the case of Frankie, a 65-year-old widow who had been living with diabetes for over a decade. Over the past few years, she had been unsuccessfully battling with elevated blood sugars and with obesity. As just one example of her daily struggle, Frankie began each day by placing a bowl of M&M's, her favorite food in the world, on her coffee table. Why? "Well," she replied, "just in case I have guests." However, as she thought back over the past year, she realized she hardly ever had guests! After dinner, she would sit down to watch TV, with her bowl of M&M's always within arms' reach, and soon thereafter the bowl would be bare. Terribly unhappy, she had convinced herself that her problem was a lack of willpower.

But Frankie had plenty of willpower. What she really needed was to clarify what was causing her werewolf eating and to develop specific strategies for overcoming those problems. Here are seven of the most useful strategies for taming the werewolf:

SEVEN SILVER BULLETS

1. Adjust your home environment to support your efforts.
2. Plan a more stimulating evening.
3. Unchain your overly restrictive daytime eating.
4. Schedule a regular evening snack.
5. Seek out alternative methods for overcoming difficult emotions.
6. Reach out to your friends and family.
7. Increase your eating awareness.

---

1. Adjust your home environment to support your efforts. Like Frankie, your most important strategy may be as simple as altering your "eating geography." If you tend to eat unconsciously while reading or watching TV, consider geographical ways to reduce those temptations. Most importantly, don't leave your favorite snack foods— like Frankie did—in such an easily available place. Put them away in your refrigerator or a cupboard, or don't buy them at all. If the werewolf emerges while you are watching TV, perhaps you could try to limit your snacking to a non-TV area, like the kitchen. Also, try some activities other than TV in the evening, like reading, walking, knitting, or making phone calls.

The strategies here are elementary: If the presence in your home of wonderful goodies is triggering your werewolf, get them out of sight or get them out of your home. If certain household activities—like TV—trigger the werewolf, consider ways to change or limit those activities. Rather than struggling with the notion of strengthening your willpower (which is all but impossible to do), start with something more sensible and straightforward—apply the simple principles of eating geography.

2. Plan a more stimulating evening. If boredom is the major trigger for your bouts of nighttime overeating, then any positive change you make needs to focus on the problem of boredom, not eating. Add some new structure to those difficult evening hours by trying a new, enlivening activity—take a walk, call a friend, take a bath, or write that letter you've been meaning to write. Most importantly, make sure that the activity that you select is not passive (like watching TV), not linked to eating, and might even be enjoyable! Going for a walk in the evening, for example, can interrupt your normal habits (like eating a bag of Doritos while reading the newspaper), take you away from the temptations of your kitchen, and stimulate your mind and body. Fighting back against boredom has helped to defeat werewolves far and wide, so give careful consideration to how you might apply this strategy in your own life.

3. Unchain your overly restrictive daytime eating. If your daylight eating is too limited, causing you to be hungry or dissatisfied by evening, then it is essential that you make some adjustments. If you are concerned about your weight, you may be frightened by this prospect, fearing that any dietary relaxation may lead to weight gain or erratic blood sugars. But this does not need to be so. For example, by consulting with a dietitian, you can experiment with ways to prevent feelings of stomach hunger in the evening. One way to do this might be to increase your intake of fruits and vegetables throughout the day, thereby increasing your food volume without necessarily adding too many calories. And if you don't eat breakfast, start.

Making changes in your daytime eating can also help to resolve the problem of eyeball hunger during the evening hours. One strategy would be to carefully incorporate small amounts of your favorite "forbidden foods," like chocolate, into your daily meal plan. Using strategies like these to enrich your daytime eating can help you to feel more satisfied and less deprived in the evening. This reduces the possibility that any hunger-related urges will lead to the emergence of the werewolf.

4. Schedule a regular evening snack. It is a terrible dilemma. Many people have found that the more they try to avoid nighttime eating, the more insistent the werewolf becomes. If this sounds like you, the best solution may be to find a way to compromise with these difficult urges. If the werewolf is continuing to visit you every night, despite all of your best efforts, then try this experiment for at least seven nights in a row (unfortunately, one night won't be enough): Plan an enjoyable and satisfying snack each night, at a time shortly before you might start overeating. And make sure that your snack is satisfying. If you typically gorge yourself on ice cream each night, don't expect that the werewolf will be satisfied with a compromise snack of carrot sticks! A better compromise is necessary. To be careful, you might want to talk to a dietitian about adjusting your other meals accordingly.

Veronica decided to give this strategy a try, treating herself to a few of her favorite cookies each evening. Because she scheduled this early in the evening, before the werewolf appeared, she did not feel as ravenous as she typically felt in the face of such "forbidden foods." By giving herself permission to do this, which was a very difficult thing for her to do, she was delighted to discover that she was less hungry, more satisfied, and less anxious during the remainder of the evening. Consequently, she was able to skip her typical werewolf snack, which usually included whole *boxes* of cookies, plus pie and cake.

5. Seek out alternative methods for overcoming difficult emotions. If anxiety, anger, sadness, or other difficult emotions serve as the trigger for werewolf eating, it is important to pay attention to those feelings as they develop and to courageously explore the real stresses that lay behind those emotions. One of the best ways to do this is to talk over your feelings with a close friend. By following this strategy, you are more likely to stumble upon a truly effective way to resolve those feelings, rather than just smothering them in food.

Veronica, for example, found that this worked well for her. After discussing the details of her feelings with her best friend one night, she realized that her familiar feelings of anxiety would begin each evening shortly after her husband would finish dinner and then sit down to read the newspaper. As the evening wore on, and he would continue to ignore her, she would begin to think about how lonely and unhappy she was in the marriage. A swirling brew of emotions would begin to build and, soon thereafter, the werewolf would begin to prowl the kitchen. Finally realizing the source of her anxiety, Veronica decided to confront her husband. After a difficult but heartfelt conversation where each shared their feelings and needs, the quality of their evenings together improved dramatically. Not surprisingly, Veronica's anxiety all but vanished and her nighttime overeating became a much rarer occurrence. So by making the effort to understand the difficult feelings that drive you to eat, you can begin to devise more effective ways than werewolf eating to soothe yourself and to resolve difficult emotions.

6. Reach out to your friends and family. In most cases, werewolf eating occurs in private. And it is a lonely experience. Overcoming this torturous habit on your own is difficult, especially when you are trying to make new changes in your life, such as taking a walk, adjusting your eating patterns, or shifting your eating geography. How could you make use of a friend or family member to support your efforts? Perhaps you would be more willing to take a nighttime stroll if you had company. Perhaps you could be more successful at quitting your TV snacking if your spouse would also agree to do so. Perhaps the werewolf could more easily avoid all those ice cream sundaes if you didn't feel responsible for keeping the freezer stocked with ice cream for the children. Explain to your loved ones that you are preparing to take some positive actions and you need their help and support. If you are worrying about imposing on them, remember that most of the changes that you want them to support—more exercise, less mindless snacking, less junk food, and more—will be good for *their* health as well!

7. Increase your eating awareness. It may sound strange, but learning how to enhance your enjoyment of food is a powerful strategy for overcoming the problem of overeating. When I first mention this to my patients, most of them think that I'm crazy. "If I enjoyed cookies any more than I already do," a typical response goes, "I probably wouldn't be able to stop after just one box! Things would get even worse!" The truth is, however, that werewolf eating is usually so hasty, erratic, relatively unconscious, and so immersed in guilt and anxiety, few people are truly aware of what they are eating.

Frankie, for example, could devour a huge bowl of M&M's during an evening, but her attention was usually on the TV, not on her consumption of M&M's. When she began to limit her M&M's to the kitchen table (following the "eating geography" strategy) and focused her full attention on this sensory experience, she found that she enjoyed them much more but—surprisingly—became satiated after only a few handfuls! In other words, by paying close attention to what she was eating, she began to automatically notice and respond to her body's subtle signals of fullness and satisfaction.

As an experiment, bring your werewolf's favorite food to a quiet, restful place. At the first try, it would be best not to do this in the evening (when you are most susceptible to bingeing). Avoid all other distractions, so don't read, listen to music, watch TV, or have a conversation. Sit down! Attend as closely as you can to the sensory qualities of what you are eating. You might even want to close your eyes with each bite. No need to enjoy or hate what you are eating; just taste it as deeply and fully as you can. And that's it!

Try this eating experiment for at least 10 minutes, 5 days in a row, and see what happens. Does something about this exercise seem unusual? Yes, I am recommending that you eat some of your favorite foods, even though they may be candy or cookies and may negatively affect your blood sugars. However, as a victim of the werewolf syndrome, you are likely to be eating these foods anyway, and in a much more frantic fashion. Since you probably realize that you cannot successfully use simple willpower to overcome the werewolf, why not try the experiment of eating your favorite goodies in a different and more mindful manner? To be careful, consider talking to your health care provider about adjusting your medications and meals accordingly.

A WEREWOLF NO MORE

Now that you know about the werewolf, you can see what a wonderful excuse he can be. When your spouse confronts you in the morning, demanding to know why the cookie jar is now empty and the bags of chips seem to be gone, you can honestly respond, "It wasn't me, honey. It was a terrible werewolf that barged in here and ransacked the kitchen. I saw the whole thing. It was terrible!" As you can see, however, much more is possible. Though battling the werewolf is difficult, he can be overcome.

Using the seven strategies, Veronica succeeded by adjusting her food choices and meal plan so that her meals were more personally enjoyable (while still quite nutritious), incorporating a tasty snack into her evenings, and resolving her nighttime feelings of anxiety by confronting her husband about her frustrations. As her nighttime overeating became more and more infrequent, she found that her blood sugars improved significantly as well. Now feeling more in control of her health and her diabetes, her mood brightened and her whole attitude toward diabetes became more peaceful.

Frankie was able to overcome the werewolf as well. The M&M's were removed from her coffee table, she faithfully practiced the eating awareness exercise with all of her most tempting foods, and she asked a neighbor to start an evening walking program with her. With a marked reduction in the number of extra calories consumed each night, her blood sugars and weight began to slowly drop, and her energy level and mood began to rise.

So make the effort to overcome your own werewolf. By identifying the specific factors that contribute to your nighttime overeating, by refusing to blame yourself any longer (remember that this is not about a lack of willpower), and by initiating thoughtful action (one or more of the seven strategies), you can succeed!

CHAPTER 6
Muddling by with Diabetes Medications

After several years on oral medications for his type 2 diabetes, Dwight listened politely as Dr. Smith explained to him that his blood glucose levels were continuing to rise and that it was necessary to begin insulin treatment. Dwight was surprised and disappointed, but he agreed to give it a try. Dr. Smith demonstrated the procedure by drawing up a small amount of insulin and injecting it into an orange, which he then had Dwight practice as well. He explained how much insulin should be administered and at what times, which Dwight assured him he could easily handle.

When Dwight returned for a follow-up visit a month later, Dr. Smith was astonished to discover that Dwight's blood glucose levels were averaging over 400 mg/dl. What on earth had happened? Dwight explained that he had been faithfully following his doctor's instructions and could not explain these shocking results. "What exactly are you doing," asked Dr. Smith. "Just like you showed me, doc," responded Dwight, "I draw up the appropriate amount of insulin at the appropriate times each day, inject it into the orange, and then eat the orange. And by the way, I'm getting really tired of oranges!"

DWIGHT'S FIRST LESSON: THE MOST CRITICAL ELEMENT OF GOOD DIABETES CARE

This story highlights several important lessons. First, all aspects of your diabetes regimen are not created equal. Although regular exercise, healthy eating, frequent self-monitoring, and regular visits to your health care provider are all vitally important, there can be no doubt that, in most cases, proper use of your diabetes medications—pills as well as insulin—will have the most powerful and far-reaching impact on your blood glucose management. It is unlikely that there is any other single action you can take that will so strongly influence blood glucose levels. Although mistakes like Dwight's are rare, many people do not take their medications as directed. In most cases, the result is high blood glucose levels, which can be disastrous.

Taking your medications regularly is not only the most important self-care task, it is also the easiest. It is much easier than making time for exercise, following a healthy meal plan, or monitoring your blood glucose regularly. However, as you know, just because it is relatively easy doesn't mean it is fun. It takes effort to remember to take your medications each day and at the appropriate times. For many people, this becomes almost automatic and painless, but for others this can be an ongoing hassle. When such feelings cause you to become lax about taking your medications, big trouble is likely. Because if you are looking for a quick and easy way to hurt yourself, there is no doubt that frequently skipping or forgetting to take your medications is the best way to raise your blood glucose levels.

How widespread is this problem? Well, not very. This is a sizable problem in certain subgroups of patients, but overall the news is pretty good:

■ In almost every survey conducted, patients report following their diabetes medication schedules much more successfully than any other aspect of their diabetes regimen.

■ In our own recent surveys, my colleagues and I found that the vast majority of insulin users (95%) take their recommended insulin doses all or most of the time. A similarly large percentage of oral medication users (94%) reported taking their pills all or most of the time.

■ Even among those patients with the most severe forms of diabetes burnout, it is not uncommon to see that they continue to take their insulin or oral medications regularly, year after year, even though all other aspects of the regimen are being ignored.

So who exactly are those relatively few people who are struggling with their medications?

Insulin Users

Among insulin users, problems are most commonly seen in young women with type 1 diabetes. In this group, more than 10% tend to cut back on their insulin, taking smaller amounts of insulin at times than recommended or eliminating some shots completely. This can also occur in men, in older people, and in those with type 2 diabetes, but much more rarely. While only a small *percentage* of people with diabetes regularly take less insulin than they should, we are still talking about a far from insignificant *number* of people—certainly many thousands are struggling. And the consequences are likely to be very severe, including blood glucose levels that are constantly high and the early development of long-term complications.

Why would anyone cut back on their insulin dosage? There are three major reasons:

1. Weight management. Without insulin, the body absorbs fewer calories from food. Thus, it becomes significantly easier to manage, or lose, weight. Unfortunately, this is truly a bargain with the devil. Weight loss may be easier, but much higher blood sugars are a guaranteed result. And these high blood glucose levels lead to long-term complications. Research suggests that those who regularly omit insulin may be at double or even triple the risk for developing long-term complications such as eye and kidney disease. Tragically, many people with type 1 diabetes—especially young women—fall headlong into this highly destructive behavior, struggling toward the temporary goal of a better figure while trading away their future health. If this is a concern for you, please see the box on eating disorders in chapter 4.

2. Fear of hypoglycemia. Many people who have had unpleasant experiences with low blood sugars become overly worried, fearful, and vigilant against the possibility that it will happen again. Cutting back on recommended insulin may decrease their risk for further hypoglycemia, but the price they pay is high. Once again, chronically high blood glucose levels dramatically increase the risk of long-term complications. If fear of hypoglycemia is a concern for you, please read chapter 17.

3. Needle phobia. Though relatively rare, a fear of needles can make each and every insulin injection a very unpleasant struggle. Individuals with this problem may tend to skip or delay insulin injections, again leading to higher blood glucose levels. If this is a concern for you, please know that there are behavioral treatments available that can help you resolve this fear. One of the best approaches is known as "systematic desensitization," which has been used successfully with many patients (including my own). Using this technique over a series of four or five visits, the individual gradually learns to associate the needle with a feeling of relaxation, rather than anxiety. Almost automatically, the fear is soon all but gone. It may seem impossible, but it really works! Talk to your doctor about how to locate a competent mental health provider who is skilled in this procedure.

Oral Medications

Among users of oral medications, the biggest problem appears to be missing an occasional pill. Nothing sinister or terrible is involved; the most likely reason is simple for-getfulness. Pills are more likely to be skipped when you must take pills several times a day. For those who take their medications only once a day (usually in the morn-ing), problems are relatively rare. However, many of the sulfonylureas and newer oral medications must be taken twice daily, and others, like Acarbose, need to be taken before each meal. In cases like these, it is much easier to forget one of your many pills, especially if you are not well organized, if your schedule changes from day to day (because of frequent traveling, for example), or if you do not have a fixed daily schedule (perhaps because you are retired or unemployed). Many people solve this problem by buying a plastic pillbox with slots for the pills to take each day of the week. One look and you know whether you've forgotten to take one.

The best solution to forgetfulness is to "anchor" your pill taking to other daily activities. For example, when he started keeping records, Rob realized that he was forgetting to take his evening oral medication at least twice each week. No wonder he was having trouble with high blood sugars! To solve this problem, he began to leave his pillbox on the dining room table (rather than in the medicine cabinet, where it was easy not to notice it during the afternoon and evening), and he promised himself that he would take his medication before dinner each evening. This worked well. By leaving his pills in a visible place and by connecting his evening pill taking with a previously established daily habit (eating dinner), he created a new daily ritual. Soon he was no longer missing any of his evening pills. So think creatively about how you can link your pill taking to other daily habits.

Sometimes the reason for missing pills is not simple forgetfulness. For example, you may be less dedicated to taking your medication faithfully if you are significantly depressed. If you suspect that depression is a problem, please see chapter 11. Another possible reason for missing pills is medication side effects. For instance, if your medication causes stomach or intestinal upset, it may become so uncomfortable that you decide to cut back on your pills. If you are having trouble with side effects, talk to your health care provider. There are many new medication choices, and your provider should be able to adjust or change your medication to minimize any side effects you are having.

DWIGHT'S SECOND LESSON:
THE SWITCH TO INSULIN ISN'T EASY

Like Dwight, many people with type 2 diabetes find the switch from oral medications to insulin to be difficult. However, unlike Dwight's problem with technique, the major problem for most people is usually emotional. In fact, many people believe insulin to be so scary and terrible that when insulin is first suggested, they refuse to take it: "Go on the needle? Not me, no way." To delay the use of insulin, they may try to bargain with their physician ("Just give me a few more months to lose some weight, OK?") or—even worse—decide to avoid any further medical visits altogether. Of course, as the delay continues, high blood glucose levels are causing more and more harm.

Does this sound familiar? If your doctor has recommended insulin and you are struggling with the idea, please consider the following seven attitudes and see whether any of them might explain your own discomfort with the idea of insulin.

1. **"If I start taking insulin, it will take over my life—controlling when and what I eat, what I do, everything!"** One of the most common reasons why people avoid starting insulin is the fear that they will lose control of their lives. Luckily, this fear is unnecessary. Modern insulin regimens are flexible, relatively easy to manage in almost any lifestyle, and not at all that scary. But don't just take my word for it! Talk to your doctor or the local chapter of the American Diabetes Association about meeting other people with diabetes who are taking insulin.

2. **"I've heard that taking insulin can cause *more* problems, like blindness."** There are many terrify-

ing stories out there that confuse cause and effect. For example, when faced with the need to take insulin, Kurt was reluctant. He thought about his mother, who had begun taking insulin after many years of poorly controlled diabetes. Soon thereafter, she had suffered serious vision loss and kidney damage. To Kurt, it seemed obvious that insulin had caused these problems. But Kurt was wrong about the dangers of insulin. The years of uncontrolled blood sugars caused his mother's complications, not the insulin. In reality, she had started taking insulin much too late. And the timing of her complications was merely a coincidence. Whether or not she had started insulin, they were bound to appear shortly.

3. **"If I have to start taking insulin, it means that my diabetes is a lot more serious than I thought."** Many people avoid insulin because they believe it is a good way to keep their diabetes from becoming too "serious." When you really think about it, that seems silly, doesn't it? If your blood glucose levels are high, whether you are taking insulin or not, the problem is serious and needs to be addressed. Not taking insulin doesn't make the high blood glucose less serious, it just makes it easier for you to ignore the problem. And when you begin taking insulin, your diabetes does not suddenly become more serious. Rather, you are now using a new and powerful tool to address a problem that has been serious all along.

4. **"Taking a needle? I don't think I could do it; it would just be too painful."** This is a common belief. After all, it sure looks like it must be painful (especially to those of us who have had painful experi-

ences with needles in the past). The truth is, however, that—thanks to modern technology—insulin injections are almost never painful. Hard to believe? Again, don't take my word for it. Talk to others who are taking insulin or, better yet, give it a try!

5. **"I've done everything I was supposed to do, and now I'm told I have to take insulin. That's just not fair."** Learning that you need to take insulin can be discouraging. It may feel like you have failed with your diabetes care ("If only I had watched my diet better, exercised more, or taken better care of myself..."). But this is not necessarily true. In many cases, oral medication is no longer sufficient and insulin is needed because the pancreas has finally—to use the professional term—"pooped out." The pancreas can no longer produce enough insulin, so outside help (injected insulin) is needed. And this is not your fault or anybody's fault; it is the natural course of your diabetes.

6. **"My doctor has told me I have to start insulin soon. But maybe if I'm really good now, I won't have to take it!"** For some people with type 2 diabetes, especially those who are obese, moderate weight loss and increased physical activity can lower blood glucose levels so significantly that insulin injections are not necessary. But bargaining like this is bad for your health! While you put off insulin for months or even years as you struggle with these tough lifestyle changes, high blood glucose levels can be doing a lot of damage. Instead, start insulin as soon as it is recommended so that you can keep your blood glucose in control. *Then* you can focus on losing weight and exercising more,

with the hope that this will help to reduce your body's need for insulin injections in the future.

7. **"I've heard that once you start taking insulin, you can never quit."** It is true that most people who take insulin continue to do so for the rest of their lives. But so what? Insulin is not like an addiction to heroin. You are always in control of what you are doing. If you decide that you hate taking insulin, then you can stop at any time—if you don't mind living with the complications caused by high blood glucose levels. And, as described above, some people do manage to make the necessary lifestyle changes so that insulin can be safely discontinued without a rise in blood glucose levels.

A Courageous Step Forward

If you are hesitant about taking insulin, the most important thing to remember is that you are always in control of what medications you are taking. It is important to challenge your own beliefs and knowledge about insulin, to talk to others who are using insulin, and—most importantly—to give insulin a try. Think about trying insulin as you would about test-driving a car. You are just taking it out for a spin to see if you like it. Tell your doctor that you are willing to try insulin, but only for a month. In almost all cases, you are guaranteed to start feeling much better. As your blood glucose levels drop, you will notice more energy, an improvement in your mood, and more. And you may find insulin to be much less of a hassle than you thought. But if you still don't think so at the end of the month, then feel free to stop taking it! Of course, the long-term consequences of high blood glucose levels are bad, but it is your choice to make. All I can recommend is that you give insulin a fair try.

EASY DOES IT

Please remember that taking your diabetes medication may be the single most important—and the easiest—action you can take to manage your blood sugars. If you are struggling with your insulin or oral medication, take steps to identify the underlying problem and address it as soon as possible. With care and patience, all of the obstacles can be overcome—from the small ones like forgetfulness to the big ones like being scared of taking insulin. And if necessary, don't be shy about talking to your health care provider about finding a regimen that is more convenient and comfortable for you. An adjustment in your timing, dosage, or drug type may make all the difference in how you feel about your diabetes medication. It never hurts to ask!

CHAPTER 7
Ten Good Reasons to Hate Blood Glucose Monitoring (and What to Do about Them)

Randi was 18 years old when we first met. She had already had a very tough life. She had been in and out of foster homes for most of it and had been living with type 1 diabetes since age 6. Diabetes had always been frustrating for her. To make matters worse, she had been struggling with an irregular eating schedule, frequent binge eating, and an inability to lose weight. She rarely checked her blood glucose, and she only took insulin when she began to feel sick. Randi had been hospitalized with diabetic ketoacidosis (DKA)—a serious side effect of high blood glucose levels in people with type 1 diabetes—14 times!

Her health care providers had always assumed that Randi was "in denial" about her diabetes, but this wasn't really true. She would have month-long periods when she managed her diabetes well, taking her insulin at the right times and checking her blood glucose frequently. These periods never lasted, however. Whenever something would go wrong (a high blood glucose reading, for example), Randi would quickly become discouraged. She was eager to be on track with her diabetes, but just didn't know how to get there.

We agreed that regularly checking her blood glucose was one of the first things Randi needed to do to get started. Randi was hesitant to begin, but she wasn't sure why. I asked her to go home that night and consider what was standing in her way. She didn't find an answer on that first night, but she was able to capture her dilemma in a poem:

> I can ride on a bike,
> do my homework each night,
> but when it comes to my health,
> I put up a fight.
> For something so small,
> just a moment or two,
> why is poking my finger
> so hard to do?
> I do things for others
> and take orders galore,
> so why is this small task
> such a big chore?
> . . .
> Oh blood sugar, blood sugar,
> come out and play,
> let's stop this fight
> and be 80 all day!

WHO DOESN'T MONITOR?

In all likelihood, your own battle with diabetes and with blood glucose monitoring probably hasn't been as dramatic as Randi's. But the feelings may sound familiar. Oddly enough, checking blood glucose is now so quick, easy, and relatively painless—and the information you can obtain is so valuable—it would seem that everybody would be monitoring regularly. Unfortunately, this is far from true. If you don't check your blood glucose as often as you should, you aren't the only one.

- Many people never check. As described in chapter 1, an American Diabetes Association survey found that 21% of adults with type 1 diabetes *never* checked their blood glucose. Of those with insulin-treated type 2 diabetes, 47% never monitored. And among those with type 2 diabetes who were not using insulin, 76% never checked.

- Many people check less frequently than recommended. In two recent studies, my colleagues and I found that approximately one-quarter of patients with diabetes do not regularly follow their doctor's recommendations for monitoring. To be specific, they check less than half as often as suggested.

It's also true that many people may fib about their blood glucose readings. Doctors have long suspected that at least some of their patients were lying about their blood sugar readings, working creatively the night before their appointments to fill their daily logbooks with "good" numbers. Of particular suspicion were those patients with spotlessly clean logbooks, where blood had never soiled a single page. But are these misgivings justified? Well, many years ago, a small group of adults with type 1 diabetes were invited to participate in a simple experiment. They were asked to follow their usual self-care over a 2-week period, checking their blood glucose at least four times daily and recording these results in their personal logbooks, but with one small change. They were asked to put aside their own blood glucose meters and to use a new one provided by the research staff.

Most of the subjects cooperated magnificently. At the end of the 2 weeks, they returned the new meters and their completed logbooks. However, what they had not been told was that these were some of the first meters *with an internal memory*. The real purpose of the study was to compare what these subjects had recorded with what the meters had actually measured. As it turned out, approximately three-fourths of the subjects were making up blood sugar readings. In fact, 40% of the logbook blood glucose levels were made up. And, not surprisingly, the majority of those fantasy blood glucose levels were significantly lower than their actual blood glucose readings.

WHAT'S SO TOUGH ABOUT MONITORING?

So we know that many people struggle with blood sugar monitoring. Some, like Randi, stop checking altogether. Many people do monitor, but not often enough to help manage their diabetes successfully. And some people fib, maybe trying to fool their doctors or perhaps trying to fool themselves. How could this be? If monitoring is so easy and valuable, why should so many people find it difficult? Is it a lack of willpower? A deeper psychological problem? As it turns out, the answer is more straightforward: people act as reasonably as possible. They stop checking their blood glucose levels or recording them accurately when they begin to believe that the whole process involves a lot of hassles and few benefits. These beliefs can be subtle. People may not even be aware of having them. But beliefs have a powerful influence on motivation and behavior. And unfortunately, blood glucose monitoring hassles abound. There seem to be lots of good reasons—some big, some small, and some silly—

to hate checking your blood glucose. Here are the top 10:

1. Your meter makes you feel bad about yourself. I have met many people who have realized, to their dismay, that their meters have become the way they judge their self-worth as human beings. Depending on their blood glucose results, they end up feeling either like a good person or like a terrible person. Does this sound familiar to you?

When you see a high blood glucose reading, do you realize that it is just a number? At times like these, many people seem to imagine that their meter is speaking to them, "What did you do wrong this time?" or "Another high blood sugar!? You are such a loser!" They are no longer aware of the actual reading, nor are they considering what action they can take. Their ability to be good problem solvers seems to vanish. Instead, they just feel bad about themselves. They may have had a terrific day in all other ways, but one unwanted number can ruin it all.

Part of the trouble is that blood glucose monitoring is often referred to as "testing." And words are powerful. If it is viewed as a blood sugar "test," this can be a subtle encouragement to consider the resulting number as a grade. You have either passed or failed. If you have high blood glucose levels frequently, this could become a big problem. Your meter may now seem like a critic who is constantly telling you that you are a failure. Not surprisingly, you may soon want to end this relationship. One of the most common ways to do this is to put the meter away in a drawer where it can't make you feel bad anymore.

2. Monitoring seems pointless (because you believe there is nothing you can really do about your blood glucose

results anyway). Imagine how frustrating it would be if you were extremely overweight and your doctor's major recommendation was that you look at yourself in a full-length mirror three times a day. How aggravating! This wouldn't help you to lose any weight. Many people think about blood glucose monitoring in the same way. As Mel and many of my other patients have said to me, "Why bother checking? It's always high anyway!" This makes some sense. If you don't know how to use this information to make positive changes in your life, then it is easy to believe that the whole monitoring process is a big waste of time. This is especially frustrating if you've been working hard to manage your blood glucose and you are still getting crazy results, blood glucose levels that seem to rise and fall for no reason whatsoever. At times like these, it seems almost sensible not to bother checking at all.

3. Checking your blood glucose reminds you that you have diabetes, which is something you'd probably rather not think about too much. No one wants to worry about their diabetes all the time. However, some people feel so upset about living with diabetes that they work hard to avoid ever thinking about the illness. This can work fairly well, as long as they don't check their blood glucose. Unfortunately, the act of monitoring can become an in-your-face, grim reminder that "yes, you still have diabetes." Far from being able to use the blood glucose information as a means to manage diabetes more successfully, they view it simply as irritating and unwelcome feedback. If they can avoid monitoring, it is possible to go for many hours without having to think about diabetes at all.

4. Your meter seems to control your life, telling you what you can and cannot do. It may seem reasonable to stop monitoring if you are feeling constantly pushed around by your meter. For example, some people report that they don't like to check before meals because a high blood glucose reading makes them feel that they cannot eat as much as they really want. For those who are concerned about hypoglycemia, a low blood glucose reading immediately before exercising means that they cannot exercise; a low blood glucose before driving means that they should not drive (at least not immediately). So, they begin to see their blood glucose results in an unusual way. Rather than seeing these numbers as simple information on which they can take some corrective action, they see these readings as commands from their meter that limit their freedom. And few grown-ups like to be told what to do, especially by some puny little machine.

5. Monitoring serves as an opportunity for your friends and family to bother you. If diabetes is a private matter for you, then frequent monitoring (especially if done in public view) could lead to conversations that you would prefer to avoid. I have seen many patients over the years who have been reluctant to check regularly because they feared that their loved ones would begin to "butt in" on their diabetes management. For example, they worried that their friends and family would blame them ("You obviously did something terribly wrong! You're probably eating too much"), offer stupid advice ("Y'know, this wouldn't happen if you'd just develop some willpower!"), or worse (see chapter 14 on the Diabetes Police for more details) if they saw a high or low reading. If you worry that regular monitoring will lead to bad feelings at home, a loss of personal control over your own diabetes care, or family arguments, then it would seem almost reasonable to avoid checking your blood glucose as much as possible.

6. None of your health care providers ever do any-thing with the results anyway. Some people have learned to use their blood glucose readings to fine-tune their diabetes self-care. Using this simple feedback on a day-to-day basis, they are able to achieve fairly stable and close-to-normal blood glucose levels. Unfortunately, many people only monitor and record their blood glucose so that their doctor can evaluate their status and recommend changes. They never learn to do it for themselves. And this becomes a problem if the doctor isn't actively involved in using this information and providing feedback. If your doctor doesn't bother looking at your blood sugar records at all, or if he examines them only superficially ("Hmmm, nothing really interesting here, so let's just keep observing your sugars over the next few months and see what happens"), why would you keep monitoring?

7. Checking blood glucose sometimes hurts. Yes, it's true that recent technological advances (slimmer lancets and a laser lancet, for example) mean that there is much less pain associated with monitoring than ever before. If you're checking correctly, it should be relatively painless most of the time. However, there are those occasions when you will strike a tender spot, and it will hurt. (Tip: If it hurts most of the time, remember to prick the sides of your fingers, where there are fewer nerve endings, not the central pads, where there are lots of nerve endings.) If you check your blood glucose a lot, your fingers can get sore or irritated, especially if you get dirt in those teeny holes. And even the sight of those little puncture marks can be aggravating. One of my patients described himself as the "Human Watering Can." He imagined that he should be able to drink a large glass of water, hold his hands above his favorite plants, and watch the water sprinkle out in a nice fine mist through his many little punctures.

8. Monitoring can be inconvenient. Monitoring equipment is small, and growing ever smaller, but if you need to check when you are out of the house (say, before dining out), you still have to remember to bring the darned thing with you! Planning is sometimes necessary, and forgetfulness is a major reason for not checking blood glucose at the appropriate times. Monitoring can take time (though not much) and may require you to interrupt what you are doing. If you are out in public and you want to check your blood sugar in private, you have to find a place to do so. This may not be easy. The perfect image of inconvenience may be sitting in a bathroom stall while precariously balancing and using your monitoring equipment. And if you're in a hurry, you can be certain that this will be that unusual occasion when your meter will somehow malfunction, requiring you to check again, and that your finger will not stop bleeding. If you believe that monitoring is a big nuisance in a life that is already trying enough, then it may be difficult to convince yourself to check your blood glucose regularly.

9. Monitoring can be expensive. If you don't have good insurance, then you probably know that regular use of test strips can be costly, especially for those who check many times each day. I remember a frustrated endocrinologist referring one of his patients to me because she was "non-compliant" with his request that she monitor her blood glucose regularly. As I soon discovered, Sarah didn't need to see a behavioral specialist like me; she simply couldn't afford to check as frequently as necessary. You can see how this could be particularly bothersome when this problem is combined with one or more of the hassles described above. For example, if you feel that monitoring is essentially pointless ("It's always high anyway!") AND it's costing you several dollars a day to be reminded of this fact, then it is even less likely that you would be willing to continue with frequent checking.

10. Life is too busy and demanding to take the time for regular monitoring. For many people, the idea of monitoring blood glucose regularly seems simple and reasonable at first. Then they are forced to juggle this task with the many other demanding tasks and stresses of daily life. Check before dinner each evening? An excellent idea, but if you're the one responsible for making dinner while also keeping your young children amused, everyone wants to eat as soon as possible, and you're very hungry RIGHT NOW, then maybe—even though your intentions are good—you just won't find the time to check this evening. In other words, life gets in the way. Perhaps you're too tired at bedtime to check or too busy at work today. Concerned about hypoglycemia, you promised yourself you'd check before you drove away from the office this afternoon, but you were already late for your next appointment. With all the other demands on your time, it is easy to become resentful about monitoring. And it's not fair, no one else has to do it! Sure, it doesn't really take very long to check. But if it interrupts the flow of your other activities, then sometimes it may seem simpler to just not do it at all.

WAIT, DON'T STOP NOW!

Now that you've read through this list, you may be even more discouraged than when you started. Even those of you who have always monitored regularly may now be ready to stop doing so. This is certainly not my intent! In fact, the good news is that each of these barriers to blood glucose monitoring can be overcome. Most people will never decide that regular monitoring is great fun, but neither does it have to be such a burden. So what to do?

First, let's be clear about the powerful benefits of regular monitoring. To date, the research results are overwhelming:

- Checking your blood glucose regularly can help you manage your diabetes much more effectively. This can help you to feel physically better almost immediately and well into the future.

- Regular monitoring can give you a wider range of options regarding food, medication, and activity. You can experience a much greater sense of personal freedom.

So monitoring is well worth doing, if only the barriers that lie in the way can be removed. So consider which of the 10 reasons, or barriers, may apply to you and let us review the four major strategies for overcoming them:

1. Have a serious talk with your blood glucose meter—especially if your monitor makes you feel bad about yourself (reason 1), you'd rather not be reminded that you have diabetes (reason 3), or your meter seems to control your life (reason 4). It is evident that many people have developed an unfriendly relationship with their meter, a relationship that is working against them. Now this may seem silly to you—after all, it's just a little machine—and you may not have even considered that a relationship of any sort existed, but clearly it does. How do you end this antagonism? How do you befriend your meter? The most important job will be to challenge your normal way of interpreting what your meter says and to realize that your meter does not have to be your enemy. Remember that there are no "bad" or "good" blood glucose readings, and *you cannot fail*. In all cases, the reading is just a number. This can be tough to keep in mind, especially if you've also had years of comments from friends, family members, and perhaps even doctors that one particular reading is "terrific" and another is "terrible."

People who are successful with monitoring view their readings as simple pieces of information and an opportunity for taking action. They may be aggravated by a high blood glucose level at first, but aggravation quickly turns to action. Think of the gas gauge in your car. When it nears empty, do you avoid looking at it? Do you yell at yourself for being so stupid as to allow it to get this low? Do you feel like a failure because you've allowed this to happen? Do you resent your car because now you must stop for gas? Probably not. You don't tend to think of the amount of

---

FOUR STRATEGIES FOR OVERCOMING BARRIERS TO BLOOD GLUCOSE MONITORING

1. Have a serious talk with your blood glucose meter.
2. Be reasonable about blood glucose expectations.
3. Learn to make good use of blood glucose information.
4. Make your environment work for you.

gas in your tank as "good" or "bad"; the gauge is just providing information that allows you to make the best possible decisions. And this is exactly the mindset to use with your blood glucose meter. But how?

First, stop referring to the process as blood glucose "testing." Instead, think of it as "monitoring" or "checking." Once you stop viewing this as a test, you will be less likely to see your readings as "grades." Also, stop referring to readings as "good" or "bad." Instead, think "high" or "low." This is more accurate and less judgmental.

Second, remind yourself how silly it is to let a blood sugar reading determine your self-esteem, to think that your meter is trying to control your life, or that it is tormenting you about the fact that you have diabetes. Challenge these automatic thoughts when they occur, and remind yourself that these readings are just numbers. One way to help this change process is to get silly and give your meter a name (and, perhaps, a personality): "My meter, Fred, told me that my blood sugar was 275 mg/dl this morning, and he went on to lecture me about what a numskull I am." And, if you want, argue back!

Third, respond to your blood glucose readings by thinking about what action you want to take. For example, if the number is high, rather than thinking, "How did I mess up this time?" ask, "What can I do about this right now?" By focusing on problem solving, you empower yourself. You can free yourself from self-blame.

2. Be reasonable about blood glucose expectations— especially if your monitor makes you feel bad about yourself (reason 1), monitoring seems pointless (reason 2), or your meter seems to control your life (reason 4). You may have overly harsh expectations for what you can actually accomplish. To avoid becoming discouraged, consider what a fair and acceptable range of blood glucose values for you would be. Specifically, at what numbers would you consider your blood sugar to be too high or too low? And in consultation with your health care provider, decide how often you should be within that range. Most importantly, this target must fit your current circumstances; it must be *reasonable* for you.

I have seen many patients with wild swings in blood glucose levels who had decided that their goal was to keep all readings between 70 and 120 mg/dl ("After all," they would explain, "that *is* the normal range"). But because almost all of their results were outside of this range, they felt like terrible failures most of the time. This sense of failure didn't inspire them to work harder on their diabetes management. Instead, it made them want to stop monitoring altogether. So establish clear and reasonable goals, and be kind to yourself. Remember that, despite your best intentions, erratic blood glucose levels will occur at times. Sometimes they'll be high and sometimes low. And these crazy numbers often cannot be explained (for more suggestions, see chapter 18).

3. Learn to make good use of blood glucose information—especially if monitoring seems pointless (reason 2) or your health care providers don't seem to actually do anything with the results (reason 6). Establish a clear plan with your diabetes care provider about what exactly to do in the case of high or low readings. In what situations do you adjust the amount or timing of your medications? In what situations do you change your food intake or activity level? And if your plan isn't working, that doesn't mean it's time to give up; rather it's time for a new plan!

I remember one frustrated gentleman with type 2 diabetes whose blood sugars had regularly been between 250 and 300 mg/dl for the past 6 months. Following his doctor's suggestions, he had cut back on meal portions and had been exercising frantically, all to no avail ("I followed the plan, but my blood sugars are still high all the time"). He was terribly discouraged as well as angry with himself. However, he had followed his plan perfectly. As it turned out, the plan needed to be changed. Through careful evaluation, it was determined that his current diabetes medication was not sufficient. The solution was simple: a new and more effective medication. Also, you should have a health care provider who is willing to work with you, someone who is active in giving you timely feedback and suggestions about your blood sugar results. If she can't or won't do this, you may need a new doctor.

4. Make your environment work for you—especially if monitoring seems too inconvenient (reason 8) or your life seems too busy for regular monitoring (reason 10). Sometimes the biggest barriers to regular monitoring are the little things, the hassles of daily life. Here are a few simple tips for using your environment to support your efforts.

If life is so busy that you are frequently skipping blood sugar checks, then consider "anchoring" your monitoring to other, already established habits (just as was recommended for medications in chapter 6). For example, in his mad rush to get to work each morning, Bert would often neglect to check his blood glucose. To solve this problem, he began to leave his monitoring equipment next to his toothbrush each morning (rather than on the nightstand, where it was easy not to notice during the morning rush), and he vowed to check before brushing his teeth. This worked remarkably well. By linking his monitoring with a previously established daily habit, he created a new ritual for his morning time. Monitoring soon became almost automatic. Think about how you can connect monitoring to other daily tasks.

If it is inconvenient to take along your meter on your daily travels, consider something as simple as purchasing another meter and leaving it where it may be needed most—at work, in your car, at your best friend's house. For instance, Nancy always planned to check her blood glucose in the afternoon, before she drove over to her boyfriend's house for dinner. She was so eager to get to his house, however, that she would rarely take the time to check. Then she would forget to lug her monitoring equipment with her. Therefore, she hardly ever succeeded at checking in the afternoon. This had gone on for years, even though Nancy was clearly frustrated with her own behavior. As it turned out, the solution was straightforward: She finally bought another meter and left it at her boyfriend's house. The moral of the story is that almost all forms of inconvenience can be overcome. To do this requires thinking creatively about how your daily environment can be modified to make regular monitoring easier.

MAKING PEACE WITH BLOOD GLUCOSE MONITORING

So what have you learned? Regular monitoring is important, yet for many people it remains tough. It can be burdensome when you give monitoring the power to make you feel bad about yourself, when you feel helpless to do anything about erratic readings, or when the demands of daily life intrude. The good news is that all of these barriers can be successfully overcome. And the keys are awareness and education. The first step is to take the time to identify which of these particular barriers may be keeping you from regular monitoring.

Perhaps you remember Mel, the 29-year-old carpenter whom we met in chapter 1. He insisted that diabetes was "no big deal." At our first appointment, Mel—who had been avoiding all blood glucose monitoring for years— agreed to the momentous step of checking his blood glucose while with me. After applying a blood sample, we stared quietly at the meter as the seconds counted down. And then, this big tough carpenter suddenly began to weep. As he cried, Mel talked about how deeply he had always hated monitoring. Throughout his teenage years, checking his blood sugar had been a difficult and humiliating experience, with his parents frequently berating him about unexplained high readings. And suddenly he understood how easily these old feelings could still surface. He realized that he continued to avoid monitoring because a high reading still made him feel like a failure and a terrible person. With this new awareness, Mel took the first step toward freeing himself from this burden. He began the process of regaining control of his life and his diabetes.

Armed with a sense of humor, consider how you can use the four major strategies for overcoming your own barriers—developing a new relationship with your meter (taking away its power to influence your self-worth), establishing reasonable expectations about blood glucose results, developing the knowledge and skills to actively use the numbers (in place of feeling helpless), and changing your environment to make monitoring easier to do on a regular basis. To support your efforts, you might want to enroll in a diabetes education program so that you can learn more about what to do with the blood glucose readings you get. Contact the American Diabetes Association at 1-800-DIABETES to find a diabetes education program in your area. And invest in a book such as the *American Diabetes Association Complete Guide to Diabetes* to find out even more.

CHAPTER 8
Ten Good Reasons to Avoid Exercise (and What to Do about Them)

The stationary bicycle, or exercycle, is one of the most common pieces of equipment in the American home. Like fleas on dogs, exercycles seem to be everywhere. But what exactly is the purpose of the exercycle? I am certain that a careful survey would reveal that the primary use of the exercycle in America is as a place to hang clothes. We are a country that loves to purchase exercise clothes and equipment of all types, but then never use them. When driving to the local mall, many of us will circle the parking lot, mile after mile, in search of a parking space that will minimize our "long" trek to the mall entrance.

We are members of one of the most sedentary cultures on this planet. We remain couch potatoes despite the impressive evidence that scientists have collected over the years demonstrating that regular physical activity, especially aerobic activity, has an enormous positive impact on all aspects of physical and mental health. In diabetes, there is no doubt that regular physical activity is one of the most important arms of self-care. Something as simple and easy as a daily walk can do amazing things: lower blood glucose, improve long-term absorption of insulin (which can help to end the aggravation of wildly erratic blood glucose levels), make it easier to lose weight, and improve cardiovascular fitness. There are thousands of touching and uplifting stories (many of which you may have already heard or read) about inactive, overweight, and often depressed people who have discovered the wonders of exercise. Exercise has lead to a transformation in their diabetes management, in their body shape and size, and in the quality of their lives. However, for most of us, these heartwarming stories seem to go in one ear and out the other. The majority of people in our society—including people with diabetes—remain firmly seated.

If you have diabetes and don't get enough physical activity, you are not alone. In surveys, my colleagues and I have found that

▎ The majority of people with diabetes admit that they are not getting enough exercise in their lives. Indeed, about one-fourth of our patients report that lack of exercise is a serious problem for them.

▎ A large number of people with diabetes (about one-third) rarely or never follow their health care team's recommendations for regular exercise.

▎ More than one-third of patients with diabetes never exercise. Never!

▎ Only about one-third of patients with diabetes exercise three times a week or more.

WHERE IS MY GET-UP-AND-GO?

Given its enormous value, why is regular exercise such an impossible undertaking for so many people? Perhaps the stories of Harry and Mona can illustrate some important aspects of this dilemma.

Harry's Story

Harry was 60 years old and had been living with type 2 diabetes for 5 years. He had been struggling unsuccessfully with his weight and blood glucose for all those years. He had always promised himself that he was going to start exercising someday. Unfortunately, that day had never arrived. When his doctor started him on insulin, Harry finally got worried enough to get serious. Following his doctor's recommendation, Harry purchased a stationary bicycle and began to ride it religiously. At first, he was able to ride for only a few minutes each day, but gradually his stamina began to build. He was soon riding for 20 minutes each morning. Within a short period of time, his blood glucose levels began to drop, he began to lose weight, and he noticed that he had more energy every day.

Harry was glad he was finally exercising, but over the next few months his excitement began to wear off. Slowly but surely, riding that exercycle every day was becoming increasingly boring. He tried reading while pedaling. Then he tried listening to the radio and even talking on the phone. But nothing really helped. As his boredom increased, his workouts began to seem more and more intolerable. He found himself looking harder and harder for excuses to skip his daily ride. Soon he was riding only a few times a week, and then not at all. His blood glucose levels and his weight began to rise. Harry felt terrible about giving it up, but he just couldn't find the oomph to get back on that exercycle.

Mona's Story

I felt embarrassed for Mona when we first met. All of my office chairs were armchairs, and she couldn't fit into any of them. Mona was 54 years old and weighed approximately 350 pounds. She had lived with diabetes for 15 years. Her blood glucose levels were always high, despite an enormous daily insulin dosage. And she had developed peripheral neuropathy, cardiovascular problems, and other long-term complications.

Because of her discomfort and shame, Mona almost never left her house, except to see her doctor. Aside from her husband, she no longer had much contact with friends or family members. In fact, Mona's life had become so sedentary that she hadn't even visited the second floor of her house, where her bedroom was, for over a year. Living primarily in her living room and kitchen, she passed most of the day watching television. Not surprisingly, she was considerably depressed.

Mona was also a bright lady. She was eager to regain control over her life and over her diabetes. When I asked her how she might want to begin, she said, "I know what I need to do. I need to get moving. Regular exercise is the key, both for my mood as well as my health." So, I asked, if she were to begin the following morning, what would she do? She responded, "I read all the magazines; I know exactly what I need to do. I need to walk 3–5 miles every day, and briskly. And there's just no way I can do that." Now in tears, Mona stood up and hurriedly left my office. It would be several weeks before she returned and we could begin the process of real change.

WHAT'S SO TOUGH ABOUT EXERCISE?

Like Harry or Mona, you may be living a relatively sedentary life. Perhaps you want to change, but feel unable to
do so. This is not because of poor willpower or stupidity.
Like people who are struggling with blood glucose monitoring or other self-care actions, you are probably
responding as reasonably as possible to the situation in
which you find yourself. In other words, you may understand and appreciate the great benefits of regular exercise,
but the benefits seem to be outweighed by the many hassles you believe are linked to physical activity. And, to
some degree, you are correct. There seem to be plenty of
good reasons to avoid exercise. Here are the top 10:

1. Exercise seems boring. Like Harry, many people find
that they get little pleasure or excitement from regular
physical activity, so they soon quit. That is certainly
understandable. It's easy to lose your desire to exercise
when your chosen activity seems more like a punishment
than a pleasure. Some people are able to discover joy in
exercise, such as the quiet peace and beauty of kayaking
across a mountain lake each morning or the simple delight
of feeling alive and aware of your body as you briskly walk
through the neighborhood each evening. But if you have
not been able to do this, then physical activity can start
to seem like a boring chore. This makes it more likely that
you will soon give up or perhaps never even start.

2. It's hard to find time to exercise. Without a doubt,
this is the most common reason for not exercising. If you
have a busy life with lots of responsibilities, it can be hard
to find the time—or take the time—for exercise. Indeed,

it is hard enough to find time to finish all of life's many errands every day! Tragically, many of the good things you may wish to do for yourself—to nourish your body, mind, or soul—often end up at the very bottom of your list of daily priorities. So they never get done. For example, you may have the best of intentions to take a long walk at lunch each day, but then there are always meetings to attend, work projects that urgently need your attention, friends who want to get together, and errands that you need to do. Of course, when you lament that there is not enough time for exercise, the underlying message is that exercise is not really that important. It can wait. Maybe when you finish all of your other responsibilities or after the kids move out or when you retire. Sometime next year, then you'll be able to start exercising.

3. Exercise may cause your blood glucose to go too low. After many years of living the good life of a couch potato, you finally talked yourself into joining that aerobics class down at the Y. You knew it would be good for your diabetes, and perhaps you could finally begin to lose some weight. And to your surprise, it was fun. But after the class, you soon realized that your heart was still pounding, you were sweating and shaking more than seemed reasonable, and your thinking seemed a little cloudy. A quick check revealed that your blood glucose was 45 mg/dl and still dropping. In a panic, you located a nearby vending machine and proceeded to gorge yourself on candy bars. So your reward for exercising that day was fear and discomfort, embarrassment, and—thanks to the candy bar extrava-ganza—weight *gain*. Aargh! Sound familiar?

If you are taking insulin, or even if you are taking one of the sulfonylurea medications for your diabetes, you may have experienced the aggravation of hypoglycemia (low blood glucose) after exercise. And if you have ever been through an episode like this, you know how irritating, disappointing, and even frightening it can be. Luckily, problems like these can always be resolved. However, if you don't know how, you may start to believe that hypoglycemia is a too-frequent and perhaps inevitable consequence of exercise. When you believe this, it becomes ever more likely that you will want to avoid exercise altogether.

4. Exercise may cause you too much pain or discomfort. It is not uncommon for people to experience aches and pains in their knees, hips, back, or elsewhere when they first start exercising. Even something as simple as a brisk walk around the block may be surprisingly uncomfortable, especially if you haven't tried to take one during the past few decades! Aches and pains can also occur because of arthritis, poor circulation, muscle weakness, nerve damage, or even angina. If you are not expecting such discomfort or aren't prepared for how to resolve such problems, it is awfully easy to become discouraged. You might end up thinking, "If exercise is going to make me feel worse than I already do, why should I bother?"

5. You are too tired to exercise. Feeling tired is one of the more convincing excuses for not exercising. After all, who can blame you? After a long day of work, running errands, or doing things with your children, you are probably exhausted. The last thing on earth you want to do is go out and work up a good sweat.

6. You don't have anyone with whom to exercise. Although some people like to be alone when exercising, many find it lonely. They want an exercise partner for the motivation, conversation, and companionship. If you can't easily find someone to join you, then this becomes a handy excuse for not exercising: "It's not my fault I don't exercise; I just haven't been able to find anyone to walk with me since my friend Shirley moved out of the neighborhood." In other words, it's Shirley's fault!

7. You think you're too old to start exercising. This is a remarkably common excuse. Some people feel that they are too old to exercise or perhaps just too old to make a change in their lifestyle. I have even met 30-year-olds who have lamented, "If I had just gotten into the habit of exercise years ago, then maybe I could do it now. But now it's too late; my knees always ache, and I'm huffing and puffing just taking the stairs to my office!" This sense of hopelessness can cripple your motivation to even try exercise, and it is easy to forget that change is possible—for anyone, at any age.

8. You think you are too overweight to exercise. There's no doubt about it, being overweight can make exercise more difficult. If you are significantly overweight, you may become worried about how you will look in exercise clothes or how embarrassed you will be if anyone sees you. I know many overweight people who would love to join a health club, but are too ashamed to actually go. It is a terrible dilemma: They don't want to be seen exercising in public until they lose weight, but they are unlikely to lose weight until they start exercising.

9. In your experience, exercise hasn't been worth the effort. If your previous attempts at exercise have not led to positive results or progress, then it is understandable that you might not feel inspired to try again. In many cases, people have unreasonable expectations about exercise.

I remember a young woman named Brenda who began a swimming program and, 2 weeks later, discovered that she had lost "only" 3 pounds. Greatly disappointed and discouraged, she abandoned swimming and never returned. But exercise rarely has a rapid impact on weight, so this was actually an impressive weight loss. In addition, Brenda was so worried about her weight that she couldn't really appreciate the other beneficial consequences of her swimming—specifically, her blood glucose had dropped markedly and her energy level was much better. Unfortunately, Brenda, like many of us, was impatient for a particular type of success. Anything less than a rapid 10-pound weight loss was a sign of failure.

10. You've tried and tried, but you just can't stay with an exercise program. This is one of the best, and worst, excuses for avoiding exercise. As an example, consider my patient, Ted, who had been trying to talk himself into an exercise program for years. Toward this goal, he had become fascinated with the wide variety of exercise equipment displayed on late-night infomercials. To the horror of his friends and family, he had spent an enormous amount of money on such contraptions, convinced with each purchase that *this one* would be the solution to his sedentary life. Of course, the novel glow of each new piece of equipment quickly wore off. Ted would grow disillusioned, retreating back into his inactive life. By the time we met, Ted—now considerably poorer—was feeling fairly hopeless. He was convinced that he just didn't have the personal discipline for exercise, and he saw no reason to even try again. Perhaps you, like Ted, have tried and not succeeded at sticking with an exercise program—because you injured your leg, because life became too busy, because exercise got too boring, because you lost your exercise partner, because you had too many hypoglycemic episodes, or who knows what. If this has happened to you, and especially if it has happened over and over again, it is certainly understandable that you would begin to feel defeated, believing that any further efforts directed toward becoming physically active are doomed to failure.

OVERCOMING THE BARRIERS TO EXERCISE

As you may suspect, those 10 reasons are merely the tip of the iceberg. There are *many* more reasons why people avoid exercise. Yet there are a large number of people with diabetes, young and old, who exercise regularly. And it gets even odder: Many of these people seem to be enjoying themselves! How could this be? The secret is that the benefits of regular exercise are much more powerful than most people know and that each and every one of the 10 barriers can be overcome. So how can you make this happen for yourself?

First, it is important to recognize that regular physical activity leads to overwhelming medical benefits, for people with diabetes and for everyone else. The human machine is designed to move. Regular activity promotes a healthier mind and body. When you are sedentary all the time, the mind and body begin to rot. Almost everyone knows at least one benefit of regular exercise. What is shocking is that the actual list of benefits is incredibly long. Exercise has a positive influence on almost every organ system in your body as well as most aspects of your psyche. And we are not talking about running marathons. Even a short, comfortable walk each day has benefits. Regular physical activity will—at the very least—promote:

- major psychological benefits (more energy, a more positive mood, enhanced resistance to stress and depression)
- major benefits to your diabetes management (a significant reduction in blood glucose levels, weight control, fewer swings in blood glucose levels, and thus a reduced risk of developing long-term complications)
- widespread health benefits (decreased risk for the development of heart disease, high blood pressure, high cholesterol, cancer, bone density loss, and other major illnesses)

Has this helped you get off the couch? Probably not. How can you change your way of thinking so that exercise feels like a priority in your life? For most people, the secret to beginning and maintaining a regular exercise program is not about learning the benefits; rather, it is about overcoming the many excuses that block your way. So consider which of the 10 reasons, or barriers, may apply to you, and let's review the seven major strategies for conquering them:

1. Search for physical activities that are fun, enjoyable, or rewarding for you—especially if exercise seems boring (excuse 1) or you haven't been able to stick with an exercise program (excuse 10). Exercise should not be something that feels too difficult or makes you miserable. Unfortunately, some people get locked into a very narrow range of ideas about what is acceptable as exercise. For example, "One of these days, I really have to start a regular walking program. But I detest walking, so I guess

> ## SEVEN STRATEGIES FOR OVERCOMING THE BARRIERS TO EXERCISE
>
> 1. Search for physical activities that are fun, enjoyable, or rewarding for you.
> 2. Modify your environment to make exercise as convenient as possible.
> 3. Develop a concrete plan for exercise that is *reasonable* for you.
> 4. Pay attention to the beneficial effects of exercise on your blood glucose.
> 5. Get some company.
> 6. Seek out professional advice.
> 7. Fight back against your own self-defeating thoughts.

I'll never exercise." To solve this problem, consider as broad a range of physical activities as possible and seek out several that you truly enjoy. This is, of course, easier said than done. If you have been inactive for many years, odds are good that you have *no idea* what an enjoyable form of exercise might be for you. A daily jog may sound good, but how can you really know whether this is pleasurable (or horrible) until you try it? The solution is to *seek out* a rewarding activity or to *transform* an unpleasant activity into a pleasant one.

Seeking out an activity. To find an enjoyable activity, you must rediscover your own sense of adventure. Make a list of several different types of exercise that you might possibly like (beginning with activities that you may have enjoyed in the past). Talk to your health care provider about which ones would be acceptable, then try them— for example, spend a week going for a short walk each day, then a week in a dance class, then a week of swimming, etc. This may sound like a lot of effort, but there is no other way to figure out what will be best for you. It's a lot like buying clothes: How can you know what will fit or look good without trudging down to the store and trying on a few different outfits? Allow yourself to be surprised by what you discover about your own unique needs.

When one of my patients tried this, he discovered that he hated walking around the neighborhood (week 1), hated swimming at the local Y (week 2), hated walking on his home treadmill (week 3), hated canoeing (week 4), but enjoyed walking on the treadmill at his local health club (week 5). As he thought about this, he realized that he only enjoyed exercise when he could "be around other people exercising who looked similarly miserable" (this was his odd way of letting me know that he enjoyed the sense of camaraderie at the health club).

Transforming an activity. If you want to transform an unpleasant activity into a pleasant one, you must use some basic behavioral principles. One way to do this is to link an enjoyable event with the selected exercise. For example, Harry (who was introduced at the beginning of this chapter) decided to purchase a treadmill and to use it each evening. To make this more rewarding, he agreed to walk while watching the nightly news (his favorite TV show) and not to watch this show in any other situation. Therefore, to watch his favorite show, he had to walk. Within a few weeks, he had successfully trained his own brain: Whereas he had previously looked forward to the nightly news, he now looked forward to his nightly walk as well. Another of my patients, Margaret, had a similar experience. Each time she used the exercycle at her local health club, she read her favorite magazines. She agreed to not read these magazines at any other time. By linking the exercycle with one of her more enjoyable pastimes, she found it easier and easier to travel to her health club each morning and begin her daily ride.

Another way to make an activity rewarding is to give it a purpose. If walking around the block is boring, then find yourself a destination. For example, Jim canceled his newspaper subscription and began walking to the store each morning for his paper. Madeleine would begin each morning by riding her bicycle to a local restaurant for her morning coffee. By giving their daily exercise a sense of purpose and by transforming this potentially boring experience into an outing, both Jim and Madeleine enjoyed themselves more. They also found it much easier to keep exercising year after year.

2. Modify your environment to make exercise as convenient as possible—especially if you find it hard to find time to exercise (excuse 2), you feel too tired to exercise (excuse 5), or you haven't been able to stick with an exercise program (excuse 10). Of the people who join health clubs, many drop out and resume a sedentary life while some continue to exercise at the club regularly. And what is one of the best predictors of continuing attendance? Simply enough, it's how far away from the health club a person lives. Those who live close are much more likely to keep going. This type of factor is seen in countless studies, all pointing to the conclusion that convenience is a powerful contributor to your willingness to exercise regularly—at home, in the neighborhood, at a health club, or anywhere. This doesn't mean that a lack of convenience should be an excuse for not exercising.

Rather, you can make convenience work to support your exercise plan. Consider the two kinds of convenience: *time* convenience and *place* convenience.

Time convenience. There is no *best* time to exercise. What is most important is to find the time that can best be squeezed into your own unique schedule. And you may need to experiment for a few weeks to find out when this might be. Some people feel that the only proper time to exercise is after work, in the late afternoon. But they are perpetually exhausted at that time, so they don't do it. The solution is, of course, to find another time. Some people find that exercising at lunchtime fits best for them, while others find that it is more comfortable to exercise after dinner. Exercising first thing in the morning seems to be the best time for many people. In fact, there is some evidence suggesting that those who exercise in the morning are most likely to keep at it over the long-term. Why? Because most people find fewer excuses not to exercise in the morning. As the day progresses, there are more and more tasks that fight for your time and attention. And your fatigue is likely to grow. Thus, once the morning has passed, finding the time and energy for exercise seems to become increasingly difficult. Please remember, though, that we all have unique likes and dislikes and that we are all living under different pressures. The most convenient time for you may remain to be discovered.

Place convenience. As mentioned above, the distance you live from the place where you exercise will strongly influence how frequently you do it. If the only exercise that you enjoy is swimming and the closest public swimming pool is over an hour away, it is not likely that you will be swimming very much. The solution is to find a way to make this activity more convenient (search out an available swimming pool that is closer) or try out some other form of exercise that is more convenient (walking around the neighborhood).

Think about other ways to structure your environment to make your chosen activity as obstacle-free as possible. If you are using home exercise equipment, must it be unfolded and set up each time you use it? Or can you find a place in your home for this equipment where it is already set up and ready to be used? If you have joined a mall-walking club, is the mall a long distance from your home or work? Or could you make a few phone calls to see if there is a group more convenient for you? It seems a small thing, but making small changes like these could mean the difference between exercising regularly and never exercising.

3. Develop a concrete plan for exercise that is _reasonable_ for you—especially if it's hard for you to find time to exercise (excuse 2), you fear that exercise will cause you too much pain or discomfort (excuse 4), or you think you're too old (excuse 7) or too overweight (excuse 8) to start exercising. If your expectations for yourself are unreasonably high, the only possible result is a sense of paralysis or failure. As you may remember, Mona had this problem. She felt that she should walk 3–5 miles each day, but realized that this was impossible for her. The only satisfactory solution, for Mona or for anyone, is to be kinder to oneself and to select an initial target for exercise that can realistically be accomplished. Otherwise, what's the point?

For Mona, this self-appraisal was not easy. After a lot of discussion, she agreed to walk each day from her front door, down the driveway to the mailbox, and then back to the house. Because of her poor conditioning, she agreed that she would rest at the mailbox for a few moments to catch her breath. As anyone with diabetes should do before beginning an exercise program, Mona talked to her doctor before starting this plan. He agreed that this activity would be safe, but—remarkably—he ridiculed the plan. He thought that this amount of exercise was "physiologically silly": it would have no noticeable effect on Mona's blood glucose or weight or any other relevant medical marker.

Of course, her physician was correct. But it was a realistic, achievable plan. If Mona could meet her goal—no matter how physiologically silly it might be—then she could begin to feel successful and personally competent, something she had not felt in a very long time. By following this approach, she could also build up her strength and stamina carefully.

When we met the following week, I could see in Mona's eyes that her spirit had been restored. "I made it to the mailbox and back every single day. Now I think its time to go to the end of the block and back." Well, okay! It took Mona a year of slow and careful increases to reach her goal of 3 miles a day, but she made it. As Mona's story teaches us, your first exercise target can be very small, even "physiologically silly," but taking that first step can propel you forward to greater and greater successes.

4. Pay attention to the beneficial effects of exercise on your blood glucose—this should be valuable if *any* of the excuses apply to you, but especially if you think

exercise isn't worth the effort (excuse 9). If there is one single thing that can encourage people to keep exercising, it is seeing concrete, positive results from their own efforts. Unfortunately, many of the most important benefits of regular exercise, like weight loss, do not happen very quickly. Thus, it is easy to feel discouraged. However, one major benefit of exercise that may occur rapidly is a drop in blood glucose levels. This is an enormously motivating discovery for most people, especially for those who are struggling with chronically elevated blood glucose. Even the most hopeless and cynical of my patients are impressed when they discover that something as simple as a 20-minute walk can significantly lower blood glucose.

So try this experiment: check your blood sugars before and after exercising on several occasions over the next week. The odds are good that you'll see a significant and consistent drop. If you don't, then you need to take an additional step: check your blood sugars at those same two times on several days when you are not exercising. You may see that because of the timing of medications or food, your blood glucose tends to rise during that particular time period (for example, if you are exercising immediately after lunch). Thus, if you see that your blood glucose level rises dramatically on the nonexercise day, but stays the same or rises only slightly on the exercise day, you'll know that exercise is working for you. Your glycated hemoglobin (HbA1c) should reflect the benefits of your exercise program as well. Compare your previous HbA1c (before you started exercising regularly) with your next HbA1c and prepare yourself for a pleasant surprise.

In addition, don't forget that there are other benefits of exercise that occur rather rapidly, such as an improvement in your energy level and the quality of your sleep. Paying attention to these changes, noticing as you begin to feel better and better, can also keep your spirit and motivation up (particularly if you are thinking that you are too tired to exercise).

5. Get some company—especially if you use being alone as an excuse not to exercise (excuse 6). For many people, companionship is an essential aspect of physical activity. Having a friend with whom you can walk, swim, bicycle, play tennis, paddle a canoe, or go to the health club can transform a boring activity into an enjoyable one. If you're not exercising because you don't have anyone to join you, then your priority is clear: You need to find someone! Take a risk and ask one of your family members, a friend, or a neighbor. Alternatively, it might be time to make a new friend. If you belong to a health club, start up a conversation with your clubmates or put up a sign that you are looking for an exercise partner. Check the newspaper or make a few calls to find a mall-walking club, a bicycle club, or a group that sponsors nature walks. There are lots of people out there who feel just like you do. By taking the risk to reach out and find an exercise partner (and, most likely, a new friend), you will be doing them a favor as well.

6. Seek out professional advice—especially if you think exercise will cause your blood glucose to go too low (excuse 3) or give you too much pain and discomfort (excuse 4). If exercise causes you too much pain, discomfort, or episodes of hypoglycemia, don't let this stop you cold. Aches and pains could be a sign that you are exercising too intensely, not stretching your muscles enough, or doing the wrong kind of exercise for your body.

If you have bouts of angina, loss of sensation in your feet, or other diabetes-related complications, you may have to be particularly careful or inventive about finding a form of exercise that is safe and effective. Whatever your limitations may be, there is *always* a way to creatively adapt some form of physical exercise to your life. Also, if hypoglycemia is a significant concern, then a thoughtful change in your medication or meal plan is likely to solve the problem. Talk to your diabetes care professional about solutions. And consider talking to a professional who is an expert at exercise, such as an exercise physiologist, who is also knowledgeable about diabetes. Such a professional can help you to discover what is wrong and to devise an approach toward exercise that will work better for you.

7. Fight back against your own self-defeating thoughts—especially if you think you're too old (excuse 7) or too overweight (excuse 8) to exercise, it's not worth the effort (excuse 9), or you can't stick with it (excuse 10). If you believe that you cannot exercise because you are too old or too overweight, please ask yourself this question: What evidence do you have that this is true? No matter how disappointing your past experiences may have been, the truth is that there is no one on this planet who is too old or too overweight to exercise. There are many people who are too old or too overweight to be professional mountain climbers or competitive triathletes (which may, possibly, include you), but that's not the kind of exercise we're talking about here! When you hear your mind whining in this manner—complaining about your age, weight, or previous history—challenge those defeating thoughts in any way that you can. For example, Mona ran into this very problem as she prepared for her first walk to the mailbox: "I've always failed when I've tried to start a regular exercise program; I'm too fat to be doing this." Rather than let her mind stop her again, she decided to talk back: "Okay, you sniveling little mind, you want to keep complaining about how fat we are? Fine, let's do it while we walk down to the mailbox and back!" And it worked!

THAT DOESN'T SOUND SO BAD

If you were told about a once-a-day pill that could help you sleep better, restore your energy, improve your mood, reduce your risk of heart disease, help you to lose weight, and improve your blood sugar control—all without any serious side effects—you would probably take it in an instant! Exercise does all this! Yet most people fail to take advantage of exercise because they have developed so many convincing reasons why they need not bother. Of greatest importance, they have lost the sense that exercise can be enjoyable and fun. Fun! As it used to be in childhood. And this is often worsened by the onset of diabetes. Exercise is usually viewed—by both doctor and patient—as simply one of many "self-care behaviors," just another chore to complete. The good news is that your sense of enjoyment can be restored and all of the other barriers can be successfully overcome. The keys to success are awareness and action. By looking closely at what excuses are blocking your path and by taking action to overcome those obstacles, you can change your whole mindset about exercise.

We have explored seven of the major strategies for overcoming these barriers: finding a physical activity that is enjoyable, modifying your environment so that exercise is as convenient as possible, developing a concrete and reasonable plan for exercise, paying careful attention to how exercise positively influences your blood glucose, finding an exercise partner, seeking out professional advice when needed, and fighting back against your own self-defeating thoughts. By selecting even one of these strategies, you will be taking an important step toward bringing the gift of regular exercise into your life.

CHAPTER 9
Harnessing Your Expectations: The Art of Developing Goals and Action Plans

With great zeal and the best of intentions, many people with diabetes have begun a new diet, a new exercise program, a new pledge to examine their feet every evening, or some other self-care change. Though successful at first, many of them soon find that other time commitments, old habits, life stresses, boredom, or other obstacles crowd out the new behavior. Enthusiasm wanes and soon the new diet is over, the new exercise program is abandoned, the pledge to examine their feet is forgotten. If you are one of these folks, if you have tried before to make positive changes in your diabetes care only to eventually meet with disappointment, then what you do right now is key.

If you want to be successful in managing your diabetes now and in the future, you must understand and harness the power of your expectations. The importance of expectations is addressed in the chapters devoted to eating, exercise, and blood sugar monitoring, but now it is time to take action. Remember that your diabetes self-care expectations, even if you are not fully aware of them, have a powerful effect on your behavior, thoughts, and feelings. Your expectations can help you or hinder you. By choosing your self-care goals carefully and making your plans with awareness, you can be successful with your diabetes care.

BRAD'S STORY

Brad had been living with type 1 diabetes since age 12, and not very happily. At age 37, he realized that he had been avoiding his diabetes as much as possible since graduating high school. A recent battle with his wife had convinced him that it was time to take some action, so he had enrolled in a 6-week diabetes education program at his local hospital. Though skeptical at first, he had enjoyed the program and even thanked his wife for convincing him to sign up.

When I met Brad, the program had just ended. He was enthused about getting back on track with his diabetes management. He realized that his blood glucose levels had been dangerously high for many years and that it was time to take action. I asked him about his plans for the upcoming week, and he responded excitedly that he was planning to "do everything just right." When I inquired further, Brad explained that he would begin checking his blood glucose four times each day, taking his insulin as prescribed (with careful daily adjustments), following a much healthier meal plan (while making use of carbohydrate counting), and jogging 2–3 miles each day.

There is no doubt that Brad had the best of intentions, but his goals were many and lofty indeed. The program was now over, and Brad was returning to his normal life. Before the education program, Brad's self-care had been remarkably poor. For decades, he had been taking a standard and unvarying dose of insulin twice daily (based on a physician's recommendation made 20 years earlier), eating what he wanted, and rarely exercising. He hadn't checked his blood glucose in years. And now he was planning to make rather sudden, dramatic changes in all of these habits.

One month later, Brad returned to the hospital diabetes clinic for a follow-up appointment. He looked sheepish and discouraged. After all the talk and effort, he was back where he had begun. Unable to incorporate so many large changes into his life all at once, he had soon given up altogether. His good intentions had run at top speed into the habits of everyday life, and his intentions had lost. I encouraged him to return the following week so that we could plan a more realistic, slower-paced strategy for reaching good self-care, but Brad was clearly too discouraged even to try. It would be 2 years before he returned and I had the opportunity to help him make the healthy lifestyle changes that he was longing to make.

Brad's story is not uncommon. It serves as a reminder that good intentions and willpower are not enough. It is sobering to realize that a large number of people graduate from diabetes education programs around this nation every day, enthused and full of hope, yet many will not succeed in making the lifestyle changes necessary for good diabetes care. Despite their best efforts, the demands and habits of everyday life soon overwhelm them.

The graduates who are successful have found a way to incorporate permanent healthy changes into their lives—exercising regularly, consistently following a healthy meal plan, monitoring their blood glucose on a regular basis, and more. As a result, their blood glucose levels are no longer chronically high. They usually feel more energetic and positive as well. To make such large and difficult lifestyle changes and—more importantly—to maintain those changes over the years is a remarkable achievement. How do they do it?

PREPARING A PLAN THAT REALLY WORKS

One of the major factors that seems to distinguish those who are successful from those who are not is how they set diabetes self-care goals for themselves and then develop a plan for action. Not only have they gained the necessary skills and knowledge, they have also found a way to harness their expectations. Unlike Brad, they avoid goals that are overly difficult, vague, or impractical. Instead, their plans for self-care are realistic, flexible, and achievable. Think you can do the same? Armed with information from the past few chapters, let us begin to set your self-care goals and plans.

Using the QuickPlan method, you will read through and complete three worksheets, focusing on three of the major self-care behaviors: monitoring, exercise, and meal planning. (Since taking medication is so rarely a problem, a worksheet for medication is not included.) When you are finished, you will have a concrete and personalized action plan. Please be forewarned that this task may not be as easy as it first seems. You will need to keep an open mind and take the time to reflect on your desire for good self-care and the obstacles that face you, and to choose realistic steps to take. It is entirely too easy to think about an aspect of self-care (exercise, for example) and say to yourself, "Exercise? I don't do it, because I just don't like it." You must look deeper into what really is blocking you. To help, each worksheet lists a series of possible obstacles and possible solutions (drawn from chapters 4–8). However, don't allow these lists to limit your own creative problem solving. You should carefully consider your own personal barriers to self-care and your own unique ideas for solving those problems.

A LOOK AT BRAD'S PLAN

To demonstrate how the QuickPlan method may help you, consider what happened to Brad when he finally returned, after several years, for a consultation. Take a look at Brad's completed worksheets on pages 140–146.

From his completed QuickPlan worksheets, Brad had several new behaviors to practice and he was ready to get started. With reasonable goals and a realistic action plan to guide him, he was much more successful than he had been previously. Over the course of several months, he found ways to build good diabetes care into the fabric of his daily life. Thus, by building on small successes, all of these new changes in his diabetes self-care became permanent. The secret was that he was able to compromise between his desire to manage his diabetes perfectly and his reluctance to give up his carefree lifestyle. A close examination of Brad's completed worksheets illustrates several important principles to remember:

1. Set achievable goals.
2. Take it slow and be patient.
3. Be as specific as possible.
4. Focus on immediate action.

Achievable Goals

Brad set smaller, short-term targets that were far more limited than what he actually hoped to accomplish in the

QUICKPLAN #1: BLOOD GLUCOSE MONITORING (Brad's completed copy)

1. In a typical week, how often do you check your blood glucose?
Two times/day or more___ Daily___ Most days___
Some days_**X**_ Never___

2. Would you like to be checking your blood glucose more frequently?
Yes, much more_**X**_ Yes, a little more___
No___ (if no, skip to Worksheet 9.2)

3. One month from now, if you are successful at making a positive change, what will your blood glucose monitoring regimen look like? Please describe in detail.

I would like to be checking my blood sugars three times/day *(before breakfast, before dinner, and at bedtime).*

4. To what degree might any of the following obstacles (described in chapter 7) keep you from reaching your blood-glucose-monitoring goal?

Potential Obstacles	Not at all	A little	Some	A lot
A. My meter makes me feel bad about myself.	1	2	3	④
B. Monitoring seems pointless.	1	②	3	4
C. It reminds me that I have diabetes.	1	2	③	4
D. My meter seems to control my life.	1	2	③	4
E. It allows my friends and family to bother me.	①	2	3	4
F. Doctors don't do anything with the results anyway.	1	②	3	4
G. Checking blood sugars sometimes hurts.	①	2	3	4
H. Monitoring can be inconvenient.	1	②	3	4
I. Monitoring can be expensive.	①	2	3	4
J. Life is too busy and demanding to take the time.	1	2	3	④
K. Other _____	1	2	3	4

QUICKPLAN #1: BLOOD GLUCOSE MONITORING (Brad's completed copy) (continued)

5. Over the next week, what are some concrete actions you will take (no more than three) to move you toward your monitoring goal?

I AGREE TO:

A. *Take action to overcome my monitoring obstacles* (each action is detailed in chapter 7). If none of the monitoring obstacles are rated as 3 or 4, please skip to part B.
To accomplish this, I will:

__✗__ Have a serious talk with my blood glucose meter (and stop self-blame).

_____ Establish goals for blood sugar results that are reasonable.

_____ Plan how I will respond constructively to blood sugar information. If it is high, I will…

__✗__ Change my environment to support my monitoring efforts—make it more convenient to do or remind myself to do it.

To be specific, I will
Each time I check, I will remind myself that this is just a number, not a comment about my value as a human being. I will focus on what action I should take, if any, rather than getting preoccupied with evaluating myself. To make monitoring more convenient, I will now leave my meter on the dining room table, where I can't possibly miss it when I need it.

B. *Modify my monitoring regimen as follows:* (make very certain that any monitoring plan to which you agree is realistic for you).
1. how often? *Twice a day*
2. at what times? *Before breakfast and before dinner*
3. how many days over the next week? *Seven (every day)*
4. other specifics? _____
To be specific, I will *Beginning tomorrow morning, I will begin checking my blood sugars twice a day, at breakfast and at dinner. I will do this every day. If things look good after two weeks, I will try increasing this to three times a day (checking again at bedtime).*

QUICKPLAN #2: AEROBIC EXERCISE (Brad's completed copy)

1. In a typical week, how often do you get at least 20 minutes of aerobic exercise (aside from your regular work or daily chores)?
Daily___ Several times a week___ Once a week___
Several times a month_**X**_ Less___

2. Would you like to be exercising more?
Yes, much more_**X**_ Yes, a little more___
No___ (if no, skip to Worksheet 9.3)

3. One month from now, if you are successful at making a positive exercise change, what will your exercise regimen look like? Please describe in detail, including type of exercise, location, and frequency.

   I would like to be walking one mile in the morning before I go to work (leaving the house right after I have my morning coffee, about 7 AM). I would like to be doing this five days a week (Monday through Friday).

4. To what degree might any of the following obstacles (described in chapter 8) keep you from reaching your exercise goal?

Potential Obstacles	Not an obstacle	A minor obstacle	A medium obstacle	A big obstacle
A. Exercise is too boring.	1	2	3	④
B. Too hard to find the time.	1	2	③	4
C. May cause blood sugar to go too low.	1	②	3	4
D. May cause too much pain or discomfort.	①	2	3	4
E. Too tired to exercise.	1	②	3	4
F. Don't have anyone with whom to exercise.	1	2	③	4
G. Too old to start exercising.	①	2	3	4
H. Too overweight to exercise.	①	2	3	4
I. Not sure that exercise is worth the effort.	①	2	3	4
J. Just can't stay with an exercise program.	1	2	3	④
K. Other _____	1	2	3	4

QUICKPLAN #2: AEROBIC EXERCISE
(Brad's completed copy) *(continued)*

5. Over the next week, what are some concrete actions you will take (no more than three) to move you toward your exercise goal?

I AGREE TO:

A. *Take action to overcome my exercise obstacles* (each action is detailed in chapter 8). If none of the exercise obstacles are rated as 3 or 4, please skip to part B.

To accomplish this, I will:

_____ Make a list of potentially enjoyable physical activities and try at least one.

__✗__ Work at transforming an unpleasant physical activity into a pleasant one.

__✗__ Modify my environment to make exercise as convenient as possible.

_____ Pay close attention to the beneficial effects of exercise on my blood sugars.

_____ Find an exercise partner or exercise group.

_____ Seek out professional advice.

_____ Fight back against my own self-defeating thoughts.

To be specific, I will

To make exercise as convenient as possible, I will try walking in the morning, right before breakfast. Also, I will bring my Walkman along so that I can listen to the morning news, which is one of my favorite things to do.

B. *Begin to (or increase) exercise* (make very certain that any exercise plan to which you agree is realistic for you).

To accomplish this, I will:

1. do what? *Walk*
2. how much? *One mile*
3. when? *Monday, Wednesday, and Friday morning, right before breakfast*
4. how many days over the next week? *Three*
5. other specifics? _____

To be specific, I will *Beginning on Monday, I will take a one-mile walk at about 7 AM, right after my morning coffee and shortly before breakfast, on three days during the next week (Monday, Wednesday, and Friday). If I am successful, I will plan to expand this to four days in the following week.*

QUICKPLAN #3: A HEALTHY MEAL PLAN (Brad's completed copy)

1. In a typical week, how closely do you follow a healthy meal plan?
Always___ Usually___ Sometimes___ Rarely _X_
Never___ Not sure___

2. Would you like to be following a healthy meal plan more closely?
Yes, much more _X_ Yes, a little more___
No___ (if no, stop here)

3. One month from now, if you are successful, how will your diet be different?

	Expect a big change	Expect a small change	Expect no change
A. Eat more high-fiber foods (like fresh fruits and vegetables, whole-grain breads, and dried beans)?	1	②	3
B. Eat fewer higher-fat foods (like oil, butter, nuts and seeds, ice cream, mayonnaise, potato chips, fried foods, salad dressing, and bacon)?	1	②	3
C. Eat fewer sweets and desserts (like cookies, candy, pie, cake, jelly, and regular soft drinks)?	①	2	3
D. Eat a nutritious breakfast more regularly?	①	2	3
E. Cut back on excessive snacking?	1	②	3
F. Have meals and snacks at more regular times every day?	1	2	③

4. Please describe in detail how you expect your diet will be different (include, for example, things you may start or stop eating, things you may start or stop cooking, or changes in mealtimes).
I will be eating a more nutritious breakfast each morning (cereal and fruit, rather than my usual donut). At dinner, I would include more vegetables and reduce the fat content (less cheese, less red meat). Also, I will plan a healthy snack for the late afternoon and evening, and I will limit my consumption of candy bars to only one day/week (Sundays).

5. To what degree might any of the following obstacles (described in chapters 4 and 5) keep you from reaching your meal plan goal?

QUICKPLAN #3: A HEALTHY MEAL PLAN
(Brad's completed copy) *(continued)*

Potential Obstacles	Not an obstacle	A minor obstacle	A medium obstacle	A big obstacle
A. Not sure how to follow a healthy meal plan.	1	②	3	4
B. I think I should be eating perfectly.	1	2	③	4
C. Too many temptations.	1	2	3	④
D. Too much stress or difficult emotions.	1	②	3	4
E. Eating at restaurants is too hard.	①	2	3	4
F. Takes too much time and effort.	1	2	③	4
G. Previous attempts have been too discouraging.	1	②	3	4
H. No support from family and friends.	1	②	3	4
I. A healthy meal plan is too boring.	1	2	③	4
J. Too hard to say no.	①	2	3	4
K. I tend to overly restrict my eating at times.	①	2	3	4
L. My life is too boring.	①	2	3	4
M. I often eat unconsciously.	1	2	③	4
N. Other _____	1	2	3	4

6. Over the next week, what are some concrete actions you will take (no more than three) to move you toward your meal planning goal?

I AGREE TO:

A. *Take action to overcome my meal plan obstacles* (each action is detailed in chapter 4 or 5). If none of the meal plan obstacles are rated as 3 or 4, please skip to part B.

To accomplish this, I will:

_____ Make certain that my meal plan is clear and reasonable for me.

__X__ Modify my eating environment to support my efforts.

_____ Consider a new perspective in the face of meal planning disappointments. *(continued)*

QUICKPLAN #3: A HEALTHY MEAL PLAN
(Brad's completed copy) *(continued)*

__X__   Utilize the principles of "structured cheating."

_____   Stay focused on the new habits I am starting (rather than the old habits I am stopping).

_____   Take action to overcome boredom in my life.

_____   Use assertiveness strategies to cope with tempting, unhealthy offers.

_____   Seek out alternative methods for overcoming difficult emotions (rather than eating).

_____   Reach out for better support from my family or friends.

_____   Increase eating awareness at difficult times (for instance, at meals or in the evening).

_____   If werewolf eating is a problem, plan a more stimulating evening.

_____   If werewolf eating is a problem, unchain my overly restrictive daytime eating.

_____   If werewolf eating is a problem, schedule a regular evening snack.

To be specific, I will *Each weekday morning, I will stop for coffee at the new kiosk near my office (rather than at the old coffee shop where I will be too tempted to get donuts). Instead of trying to give up sweets completely, I will pledge to have 1–2 candy bars each Sunday. Finally, I will ask my wife to purchase a big bag of presliced and prewashed mixed vegetables at the market (so it will be easier for us to include them at all dinner meals).*

B. *Modify my current meal plan as follows* (make very certain that any meal plan changes to which you agree are realistic for you):

Beginning tomorrow, I will plan to have cereal and fruit for breakfast, at least 5 mornings/week. With my wife's cooperation, I will have a vegetable dish at dinner at least 5 nights/ week. Each evening, I will plan to have a healthy snack (probably popcorn) around 9 PM. This should help me to avoid my strong evening urges for chips and crackers.

long run. For each of the self-care actions, he thoughtfully considered what he could *reasonably* change over the next month. He expected, for example, that he would eventually be checking his blood sugars at least four times each day, but he realized that it was foolish to think that he could make such a big change in his lifestyle immediately. Remember that you must temper your expectations with what you can actually do right now.

Slow and Patient

As Brad planned the specific actions he would begin that first week, he was careful to limit his changes to a fairly small number of behaviors. And this certainly wasn't easy for him. In the meal planning section, for example, he was tempted to say, "Look, I'm just going to try to eat perfectly tomorrow." It was much more difficult to select one or two actions that would help him start along the path to eating a more nutritious breakfast, dinner, and evening snack.

Concrete Actions

When Brad had completed the worksheets, he knew exactly what steps he would then take. He had planned where he would leave his meter, when he would leave for his walk each morning and where he would go, and what he would have for his evening snack the next night. For many people, well-intentioned plans often founder on the rocks of vagueness. For example, they may have vowed to exercise during the coming week, but they didn't know exactly what type of exercise they would do or exactly when they would do it. Not surprisingly, inertia sets in, and nothing gets accomplished. With a clear action plan like Brad's, the odds are much greater that you will actually follow it.

Immediate Action

After completing the three worksheets, Brad was ready to begin the selected behavior changes. Actions truly matter. By making thoughtful changes in your self-care, no matter how small or limited those changes may seem at first, you can regain a sense of control over your health and your life.

IT'S YOUR TURN

Now it's your turn to complete the three QuickPlan worksheets (9.1, 9.2, and 9.3) and set some achievable action goals for yourself. When you've completed the worksheets, close the book and try taking a few of your new self-care behaviors out for a test drive.

WORKSHEET 9.1 QUICKPLAN #1: BLOOD GLUCOSE MONITORING

1. In a typical week, how often do you check your blood glucose?
   Two times/day or more___ Daily___ Most days___
   Some days___ Never___

2. Would you like to be checking your blood glucose more frequently?
   Yes, much more___ Yes, a little more___
   No___ (if no, skip to Worksheet 9.2)

3. One month from now, if you are successful at making a positive change, what will your blood glucose monitoring regimen look like? Please describe in detail.

   _____

   _____

   _____

   _____

4. To what degree might any of the following obstacles (described in chapter 7) keep you from reaching your blood-glucose-monitoring goal?

Potential Obstacles	Not at all	A little	Some	A lot
A. My meter makes me feel bad about myself.	1	2	3	4
B. Monitoring seems pointless.	1	2	3	4
C. It reminds me that I have diabetes.	1	2	3	4
D. My meter seems to control my life.	1	2	3	4
E. It allows my friends and family to bother me.	1	2	3	4
F. Doctors don't do anything with the results anyway.	1	2	3	4
G. Checking blood sugars sometimes hurts.	1	2	3	4
H. Monitoring can be inconvenient.	1	2	3	4
I. Monitoring can be expensive.	1	2	3	4
J. Life is too busy and demanding to take the time.	1	2	3	4
K. Other _____	1	2	3	4

(*continued*)

WORKSHEET 9.1 QUICKPLAN #1: BLOOD GLUCOSE MONITORING *(continued)*

5. Over the next week, what are some concrete actions you will take (no more than three) to move you toward your monitoring goal?

I AGREE TO:

A. *Take action to overcome my monitoring obstacles* (each action is detailed in chapter 7). If none of the monitoring obstacles are rated as 3 or 4, please skip to part B.

To accomplish this, I will:

_____ Have a serious talk with my blood glucose meter (and stop self-blame).

_____ Establish goals for blood sugar results that are reasonable.

_____ Plan how I will respond constructively to blood sugar information. If it is high, I will...

_____ Change my environment to support my monitoring efforts—make it more convenient to do or remind myself to do it.

To be specific, I will

_____

_____

_____

_____

_____

B. *Modify my monitoring regimen as follows:* (make very certain that any monitoring plan to which you agree is realistic for you).

1. how often? _____

2. at what times? _____

3. how many days over the next week? _____

4. other specifics? _____

To be specific, I will _____

_____

_____

_____

_____

WORKSHEET 9.2 QUICKPLAN #2: AEROBIC EXERCISE

1. In a typical week, how often do you get at least 20 minutes of aerobic exercise (aside from your regular work or daily chores)?
Daily___   Several times a week___   Once a week___
Several times a month___   Less___

2. Would you like to be exercising more?
Yes, much more___   Yes, a little more___
No___ (if no, skip to Worksheet 9.3)

3. One month from now, if you are successful at making a positive exercise change, what will your exercise regimen look like? Please describe in detail, including type of exercise, location, and frequency.

_____

_____

_____

_____

4. To what degree might any of the following obstacles (described in chapter 8) keep you from reaching your exercise goal?

Potential Obstacles	Not an obstacle	A minor obstacle	A medium obstacle	A big obstacle
A. Exercise is too boring.	1	2	3	4
B. Too hard to find the time.	1	2	3	4
C. May cause blood sugar to go too low.	1	2	3	4
D. May cause too much pain or discomfort.	1	2	3	4
E. Too tired to exercise.	1	2	3	4
F. Don't have anyone with whom to exercise.	1	2	3	4
G. Too old to start exercising.	1	2	3	4
H. Too overweight to exercise.	1	2	3	4
I. Not sure that exercise is worth the effort.	1	2	3	4
J. Just can't stay with an exercise program.	1	2	3	4
K. Other _____	1	2	3	4

(*continued*)

WORKSHEET 9.2 QUICKPLAN #2: AEROBIC EXERCISE *(continued)*

5. Over the next week, what are some concrete actions you will take (no more than three) to move you toward your exercise goal?

I AGREE TO:

A. *Take action to overcome my exercise obstacles* (each action is detailed in chapter 8). If none of the exercise obstacles are rated as 3 or 4, please skip to part B.

To accomplish this, I will:

_____ Make a list of potentially enjoyable physical activities and try at least one.

_____ Work at transforming an unpleasant physical activity into a pleasant one.

_____ Modify my environment to make exercise as convenient as possible.

_____ Pay close attention to the beneficial effects of exercise on my blood sugars.

_____ Find an exercise partner or exercise group.

_____ Seek out professional advice.

_____ Fight back against my own self-defeating thoughts.

To be specific, I will

_____

_____

_____

_____

_____

B. *Begin to (or increase) exercise* (make very certain that any exercise plan to which you agree is realistic for you).

To accomplish this, I will:

1. do what? _____

2. how much? _____

3. when? _____

4. how many days over the next week?_____

5. other specifics? _____

To be specific, I will _____

_____

_____

_____

_____

WORKSHEET 9.3 QUICKPLAN #3:
A HEALTHY MEAL PLAN

1. In a typical week, how closely do you follow a healthy meal plan?
Always___ Usually___ Sometimes___ Rarely___
Never___ Not sure___

2. Would you like to be following a healthy meal plan more closely?
Yes, much more___ Yes, a little more___
No___ (if no, stop here)

3. One month from now, if you are successful, how will your diet be different?

	Expect a big change	Expect a small change	Expect no change
A. Eat more high-fiber foods (like fresh fruits and vegetables, whole-grain breads, and dried beans)?	1	2	3
B. Eat fewer higher-fat foods (like oil, butter, nuts and seeds, ice cream, mayonnaise, potato chips, fried foods, salad dressing, and bacon)?	1	2	3
C. Eat fewer sweets and desserts (like cookies, candy, pie, cake, jelly, and regular soft drinks)?	1	2	3
D. Eat a nutritious breakfast more regularly?	1	2	3
E. Cut back on excessive snacking?	1	2	3
F. Have meals and snacks at more regular times every day?	1	2	3

4. Please describe in detail how you expect your diet will be different (include, for example, things you may start or stop eating, things you may start or stop cooking, or changes in mealtimes).

_____

_____

_____

_____

5. To what degree might any of the following obstacles (described in chapters 4 and 5) keep you from reaching your meal plan goal?

(continued)

WORKSHEET 9.3 QUICKPLAN #3:
A HEALTHY MEAL PLAN *(continued)*

Potential Obstacles	Not an obstacle	A minor obstacle	A medium obstacle	A big obstacle
A. Not sure how to follow a healthy meal plan.	1	2	3	4
B. I think I should be eating perfectly.	1	2	3	4
C. Too many temptations.	1	2	3	4.
D. Too much stress or difficult emotions.	1	2	3	4
E. Eating at restaurants is too hard.	1	2	3	4
F. Takes too much time and effort.	1	2	3	4
G. Previous attempts have been too discouraging.	1	2	3	4
H. No support from family and friends.	1	2	3	4
I. A healthy meal plan is too boring.	1	2	3	4
J. Too hard to say no.	1	2	3	4
K. I tend to overly restrict my eating at times.	1	2	3	4
L. My life is too boring.	1	2	3	4
M. I often eat unconsciously.	1	2	3	4
N. Other _____	1	2	3	4

6. Over the next week, what are some concrete actions you will take (no more than three) to move you toward your meal planning goal?

I AGREE TO:

A. *Take action to overcome my meal plan obstacles* (each action is detailed in chapter 4 or 5). If none of the meal plan obstacles are rated as 3 or 4, please skip to part B.

To accomplish this, I will:

_____ Make certain that my meal plan is clear and reasonable for me.

_____ Modify my eating environment to support my efforts.

WORKSHEET 9.3 QUICKPLAN #3:
A HEALTHY MEAL PLAN *(continued)*

_____ Consider a new perspective in the face of meal planning disappointments.

_____ Utilize the principles of "structured cheating."

_____ Stay focused on the new habits I am starting (rather than the old habits I am stopping).

_____ Take action to overcome boredom in my life.

_____ Use assertiveness strategies to cope with tempting, unhealthy offers.

_____ Seek out alternative methods for overcoming difficult emotions (rather than eating).

_____ Reach out for better support from my family or friends.

_____ Increase eating awareness at difficult times (for instance, at meals or in the evening).

_____ If werewolf eating is a problem, plan a more stimulating evening.

_____ If werewolf eating is a problem, unchain my overly restrictive daytime eating.

_____ If werewolf eating is a problem, schedule a regular evening snack.

To be specific, I will

_____

_____

_____

_____

_____

B. *Modify my current meal plan as follows* (make very certain that any meal plan changes to which you agree are realistic for you):

_____

_____

_____

_____

_____

Feelings and Attitudes

CHAPTER 10
Worrying about Long-Term Complications: The Uses and Misuses of Fear

Let's begin with the bad news. The simple fact is that if you have diabetes, you are at higher risk than other people for the development of long-term complications, such as heart, eye, nerve, and kidney disease. Diabetes is a very serious disease. Given this information, it is understandable that you might worry about your health at times, that you might become frightened or even terrified about your future, or even that you might sink into deep despair or denial. In fact, fears about diabetes are far from rare. My colleagues and I have found that:

■ One in five of our surveyed patients report that they worry excessively about the future and the possibility that they could develop serious long-term complications.

■ About the same number feel doomed, believing that they will end up with serious long-term complications, no matter what they do.

So if you are worrying about the damage that diabetes might wreak on your body, welcome to the club!

Though fear is commonplace, it is important to emphasize that the facts about complications really aren't simple at all. Although diabetes must be taken seriously, having it does not mean that you are doomed. Far from it! And, as it turns out, three things you can control—your understanding of the real dangers of diabetes, how you make use of these facts, and how you wield the power of your own fears and worries—play a powerful role in how well you manage diabetes and how comfortably you live with the illness. In other words, you can use your fears wisely—to help you rather than hinder you.

To live well with diabetes means finding a way to harness the power of fear. This requires a delicate balancing act. The secret is being able to understand and influence your own way of thinking. How you think about diabetes will determine how frightened you are and how you are able to cope with fear. Those who are successful have found a comfortable midpoint, a point of balance between the two extremes of fear: feeling totally invincible ("The long-term complications of diabetes will never happen to me") and feeling completely terrified by diabetes ("I am doomed and there's nothing that I can do about it"). In other words, they are frightened enough to care for their diabetes, but not so frightened that they are paralyzed.

THE PROBLEM WITH BEING FEARLESS

We know that there are many people who feel invulnerable to the long-term complications of diabetes. They are fearless because they are certain that diabetes cannot harm them. From their perspective, diabetes may be serious for other people, but not for them. Their diabetes is merely "a touch of sugar." Because they feel fine and there are no obvious wounds that remind them of the presence of diabetes, it is easy to imagine that the illness is not real—at least not until the onset of complications. Other people hold a similar belief that vulnerability to complications doesn't matter. They are fearless because they think, "We're all going to die some day, so why should I worry about the effects of diabetes on my body?" If you share either of these beliefs about diabetes, then you are—of course—unlikely to feel inspired to take good care of yourself. Why should you bother?

The only problem with these ways of thinking is that they are *just plain wrong*. Whether you choose to believe it or not, diabetes can hurt you. And the major concern should not be that diabetes will kill you (since it is true that we all will die eventually), but that diabetes has the potential to ruin the quality of your life and to shorten it. To believe that you are invulnerable reflects a serious lack of knowledge about diabetes.

IS IT GOOD TO BE FRIGHTENED?

So if being completely fearless about diabetes is not a good idea, then worrying about diabetes must be good for you, right? To feel motivated, you should be terrified by the possibility of long-term complications. Correct? Well, not really. It is widely believed that one of the major reasons why many people don't take good care of their diabetes is because they just aren't scared enough. Over one-third of primary care physicians believe that if their patients really understood how harmful diabetes can be, *then* they would be motivated to manage their diabetes closely. This is probably why doctors, as well as family and friends, often make such nagging and threatening comments as:

■ "If you don't get your blood sugars under control, you're going to lose your feet."

■ "You need to start eating better or you're going to end up just like that blind patient in the waiting room."

Unfortunately, fear doesn't work as well as people think. In fact, there is no good evidence that those who are more frightened about long-term complications manage their diabetes more aggressively than anyone else. In fact, my colleagues and I have found the opposite effect: Those with the poorest self-care are somewhat more worried about complications than those with better self-care.

So why does fear motivate some people, but not others? To answer this question, consider the following stories.

Len

Len was 28 years old and had been living with type 1 diabetes for almost 20 years. He had been ignoring his diabetes for many years, and his blood glucose levels averaged close to 300 mg/dl. Therefore, I was amazed and gratified when he decided to attend the hospital's diabetes support group. During that session, all participants were asked to draw a picture of what it felt like to be living with diabetes. Len's drawing was remarkable. It was filled with syringes, foods, blood glucose meters, and irate-looking family members, but attention was drawn to a small oddly shaped, bulbous clock in the middle of the picture. As Len explained it, "This is the centerpiece of my picture: a quietly ticking time bomb. Though I try to ignore it, I know it is always there in the background, inside of me, and that one day it is going to explode. All of the terrible complications of diabetes will begin to occur, and they will eventually kill me. And there is nothing I can do about it." Len lived in terror of long-term complications, but that terror had never motivated him to take good care of his diabetes. Instead, he felt so frightened and helpless that he did his best to avoid thinking about diabetes at all. Despite his best efforts at denial, the terrible ticking of his time bomb seemed to follow him everywhere.

Bonnie

Bonnie was shocked when she was diagnosed with type 1 diabetes at the age of 24. From what she had heard about diabetes over the years, she was sure that diabetes was a death sentence. But over the next 7 years, Bonnie learned about intensive diabetes management and achieved near-normal blood glucose levels. Despite this success, she could not shake the sense of being doomed. Though she was free from complications and all laboratory test results were good, she felt certain that kidney disease was approaching. At age 31, she continued to believe that she would not live long enough to see her two young children graduate from high school. She believed that all that awaited her was dialysis and an early death. At the same time, Bonnie never wavered in her efforts to manage her diabetes as closely as possible, hoping against hope that tight blood glucose control would help her to delay the inevitable.

Nora

When Nora began to experience problems with her feet, she knew it was time to take action. She had developed type 2 diabetes many years earlier, but had never really taken it seriously. After all, she felt fine, so why should she worry about diabetes? Now, at age 60, the worsening numbness and discomfort in her legs had been diagnosed as painful peripheral neuropathy. It had started out as just an occasional tingling, but it had slowly grown more intense and more uncomfortable. Now, even the feel of the bed sheets on her legs caused her significant pain. Her doctor assured her that this would only get worse if she did not put more effort in to carefully managing her blood glucose. There would be more pain, foot problems would be more likely, wounds would not heal easily, and the possibility of amputation would greatly increase.

Diabetes was suddenly very real and very worrisome. Nora thought of her mother, who had suffered terribly because of complications of diabetes. It suddenly seemed likely that Nora was going to end up traveling the same path. Terrified by this possibility, Nora enrolled in a diabetes education program and soon transformed her lifestyle. With surprisingly little difficulty, she began exercising regularly, checking her blood glucose twice daily, and following a much healthier meal plan. She now understood that diabetes was a serious disease, and she was going to manage it as well as possible.

The Uses of Fear

Len, Bonnie, and Nora were all frightened by the prospects of long-term complications, but they responded to their fear in very different ways. What can explain these different responses to fear? The answer is simple: Unlike Len and Bonnie, Nora felt certain that she could do something about the terrible bogeyman of complications. She did not feel helpless. Instead, she was able to use her fear to improve her diabetes care. And this helped her feel more confident about her health and her future. In contrast, Len and Bonnie felt doomed. Although Bonnie kept alive at least a spark of hope that her self-care efforts might be of some value, Len felt completely powerless. As

Len's case demonstrates, fear can be paralyzing—keeping you from improving your self-care—when you believe that your actions cannot help you overcome the scary situation.

WHAT TO DO ABOUT FEAR

If you are living at one of the extremes of fear, you may be especially interested in learning how to achieve Nora's point of balance. Here are four strategies that can help you make use of your fears:

1. Explore your unconscious thoughts about diabetes and learn why they are making you feel so frightened (or so fearless).
2. Learn about the real risks of developing long-term complications.
3. When your thoughts about long-term complications become too scary, don't forget to remind yourself about the facts.
4. Learn about the powerful benefits of good diabetes care.

Exploring Your Unconscious Thoughts

Perhaps you don't think of yourself as a gambler, but you are. As you travel though life each day, you make decisions based on what you see as the risks and rewards, the odds that any action you take will be successful or not successful. Much of this thinking occurs outside of your immediate awareness. But it dramatically influences your thoughts, feelings, and actions. You are always playing the odds. For instance, how were you able to jet across the country last week, 30,000 feet in the air, without suffering a major anxiety attack? Somewhere in the deep recesses of your brain, you decided that the odds of the plane crashing were so low (much less than one in a million) that you could travel safely and without fear. Or why did you drive to the supermarket yesterday without wearing your seat belt? Once again, you decided that the odds of a traffic accident were so low that it was worth the risk.

Your thoughts and feelings about diabetes work in a similar fashion. Depending on how you think about the odds that long-term complications will develop—even though these thoughts may be mostly unconscious—you will feel invulnerable, somewhat concerned, very worried, or terrified and despairing. What do you think the odds are that diabetes will cause you to go blind within the next 20 years? What about the odds that you will suffer kidney damage, end up on dialysis, or have a significantly shorter life span than people without diabetes? Of course, you cannot know the real odds, but do you realize what you think your chances are?

Worksheet 10.1 lists just a sample of the many health concerns that worry people with diabetes. You can complete it now to find out what you believe your odds to be.

The purpose of this simple worksheet is to give you a quick peek at your hidden thoughts. So take a careful look now at your responses.

If your answers are on or near the extreme left side of the worksheet (especially for question 1), you probably feel invulnerable. You may believe that complications cannot happen to you. Like the folks described earlier, you may be in serious trouble, especially if your beliefs are causing you to be lax about your diabetes care. If your answers are toward the extreme right side of the worksheet for questions 1–3 (complications seem likely) and toward the left side for questions 4–6 (there seems little that can be done to stop or delay them), you are probably feeling doomed.

WORKSHEET 10.1: GUESSING ABOUT MY FUTURE

Please respond to each question with your best guess. There are no correct answers, so please do not worry about whether your answer is factually accurate. What is most important is to indicate as honestly as possible what you really believe.

A. What would you estimate are the chances that diabetes will:

1. Negatively impact on your long-term health?

___0 (won't happen)   ___1/1,000 (might happen)   ___1/100 (a fair chance)   ___50/50 (pretty likely)   ___1/1 (will happen)

2. Cause you to lose your eyesight?

___0 (won't happen)   ___1/1,000 (might happen)   ___1/100 (a fair chance)   ___50/50 (pretty likely)   ___1/1 (will happen)

3. Cause you to suffer serious kidney damage and end up on dialysis?

___0 (won't happen)   ___1/1,000 (might happen)   ___1/100 (a fair chance)   ___50/50 (pretty likely)   ___1/1 (will happen)

B. To what degree do you think that taking good care of your diabetes could reduce your risk of:

4. Suffering negative consequences to your health over the years?

___It wouldn't help.   ___It would help a little.   ___It would help a fair amount.   ___It would help a great deal.

5. Losing your eyesight?

___It wouldn't help.   ___It would help a little.   ___It would help a fair amount.   ___It would help a great deal.

6. Suffering serious kidney damage and ending up on dialysis?

___It wouldn't help.   ___It would help a little.   ___It would help a fair amount.   ___It would help a great deal.

Worrying about Long-Term Complications   **167**

When you have such unrealistic beliefs, like those of Len and Bonnie, it is not surprising that chronic fear and despair will follow. For example, if the odds of losing your eyesight during your lifetime really were 50/50, then feeling frightened and powerless would make a great deal of sense. However, these odds are not accurate. Will half of all people with diabetes go blind? No, far from it!

To harness your fears, you need to be aware of the truth, the real risks concerning complications and the facts about how good diabetes care can reduce those risks. Many people have come to believe in unrealistic odds about complications because the real risks are rarely publicized. And there is a tendency to manufacture your own ideas about the odds based on what you see and hear around you— from family members who have suffered severe complications to friends with long-standing diabetes who seem to be in pretty good health. By shining the light of your conscious mind on your hidden beliefs, you can begin to understand how they affect your fear of diabetes (or lack thereof). With this awareness, you can begin to question whether your beliefs are really accurate. By challenging these beliefs and by staying open to new evidence, you are taking the first steps toward harnessing your fears.

Learning about the Real Risks

If you identify with Len or Bonnie, feeling that diabetes has doomed you to a short and painful life, here is a remarkable story that may help you regain a sense of perspective. In 1980, Professor Michael Bliss, a historian at the University of Toronto, decided to research the story behind the discovery of insulin in the early 1920s. In addition to describing the scientific investigations of the codiscoverers, Banting and Best, he examined the cases of the first recipients of insulin. Dr. Banting's prize patient was a 15-year-old named Elizabeth Evans Hughes, whose father, Charles Evans Hughes, was then Secretary of State under President Warren Harding. Like most others with type 1 diabetes at the time, Elizabeth was destined to die at a very early age. Indeed, by the time she reached Dr. Banting's office in Toronto in late 1922, she weighed only 45 pounds and was close to death. However, the discovery of insulin changed everything. Elizabeth began to receive twice-daily injections of the newly discovered hormone, and under Dr. Banting's guidance, she recovered rapidly. After returning home, she kept in touch with Dr. Banting for several years, with the last letter arriving in 1926.

There was no record of what happened to Elizabeth after that, but it seemed likely that she had died shortly thereafter. After all, she was taking wildly varying doses of a brownish, impure extract of insulin mixed with God-knows-what-else, and there was no technology available for monitoring changes in blood glucose. Given such primitive conditions, long-term complications had surely arisen and Elizabeth was unlikely to have survived for very long.

Professor Bliss began to wonder exactly how long Elizabeth had lived and to what degree she had suffered from complications. In his investigation, he discovered that Elizabeth had married a prominent young lawyer in 1930 and, to his amazement, was still alive in 1948 at the time of her father's death. Professor Bliss' continuing search revealed that Elizabeth's husband was still alive in 1980. With some excitement, Professor Bliss wrote to him, inquiring about his wife's fate—when had she died and what had been the later course of her illness? To his great shock, Professor Bliss soon received the following letter in response:

Dear Professor Bliss,

Your letter of August 7, addressed to my husband was read with interest by both of us. Yes—I am very much alive, in good health and spirits and amazed that after you had read my medical record in Dr. Banting's papers, you were able to find me. Day after tomorrow will be my 73rd birthday and 58 years since I celebrated my 15th, having just arrived in Toronto to be Dr. Banting's third patient in a last-minute effort to save my life....

In an era in which many children with type 1 diabetes did not live past the age of 30, Elizabeth prospered. She lived to a ripe old age, relatively free from long-term complications and in good mental and physical health.

The point of this story? Diabetes is not a death sentence. Yes, tragedy still occurs. Some people develop long-term complications much too soon and die at a terribly young age. However, there can be no doubt that more and more people with diabetes are—like Elizabeth—living longer and healthier lives. With new medications, new diabetes technologies (such as blood glucose monitoring), and new ways to slow the development of complications, the future can only be brighter. With good care, there is no reason that you cannot live as long, or longer, than anyone else.

Remembering the Facts

Sometimes your thoughts can seem like spooked cattle. One moment they are munching contentedly in a quiet pasture, and the next moment—after a single gunshot, a simple thought—they are running in a blind panic. What causes such a "mental stampede"? I remember a bright young attorney named Frank who, at his quarterly visit to his endocrinologist, discovered that he had developed the first signs of diabetic eye disease. Up to that time, Frank had been free from complications. When I met him later that day, he was terrified and despairing, certain that he would soon be a homeless beggar on the streets, blind and legless. I remember a middle-aged schoolteacher named Nancy, whose best friend had suffered kidney failure (secondary to her diabetes) and died earlier that month. Even though Nancy had intensively managed her diabetes for many years (in sharp contrast to her friend) and there had never been the slightest trace of kidney problems, she became all but convinced that she was doomed. Even though she knew it was irrational, she became overwhelmingly frightened that her fate would soon lead her, like her dear friend, to dialysis and death.

You can fight back against these stampeding fears, just like Frank and Nancy did, by challenging your thoughts with some important facts. One set of facts that you can employ are the actual risks, but there are two other important strategies that may help:

▌ Remind yourself that one complication does not spell doom.

▌ Remind yourself that your own situation is unique.

There is no evidence that developing one complication means that you are doomed to develop others. In addition, good care can slow or halt the progression of many, though not all, complications (as Frank learned, for instance, his risk of suffering serious vision loss was still quite low, even with the development of retinopathy).

GOOD NEWS ABOUT COMPLICATIONS

When it comes to complications, scientific evidence over the past few years has shown that the actual odds can be a great deal better than you might think, especially with recent advances in early diagnosis and treatment of problems. Here are some examples of your real risks for developing serious complications.

Eye Disease/Blindness

Although mild diabetic retinopathy will eventually develop in most people with diabetes, serious vision problems are a different story. Evidence from two major studies, the Wisconsin Epidemiologic Study of Diabetic Retinopathy and the Diabetes Control and Complications Trial (DCCT), indicates that:

▮ If you are a 30-year-old with type 1 diabetes, you have an 88% chance of still having good vision at age 60.
▮ If you are a 50-year-old with type 2 diabetes, you have about a 93% chance of still seeing well at age 70.
▮ With newer treatments and technologies, your current chances are probably even better.
▮ Intensive diabetes management can reduce the risk of retinopathy by 60%.
▮ In people who already have retinopathy, intensive management can slow its progression by 55%.

The bottom line is this: In this day and age, if you participate in a comprehensive treatment program that includes intensive diabetes management and regular eye exams with a well-trained diabetic ophthalmologist, the odds that you will never experience serious vision loss or blindness are very good, probably 99% or better.

Kidney Disease

A recent study found that:

▮ After 35 years of diabetes, 21% of patients had suffered renal failure. However, this varied widely depending on long-term blood glucose control.
▮ Among people with the poorest glucose control (the highest blood sugars), about 36% ended up in kidney failure.

GOOD NEWS *(continued)*

▌ Among those with the best control (the lowest blood sugars), only 9% ended up in kidney failure.

If those odds still sound pretty bad, remember that the people in the study were diagnosed in the late 1950s— many years before the development of self-monitoring of blood glucose, new medications to protect the kidneys, and other advances in prevention and treatment.

Keep in mind that the DCCT found that intensive diabetes management reduced the risk of serious kidney damage by 56% in people with type 1 diabetes. And the same is likely to be true for people with type 2 diabetes. When you manage your diabetes carefully, working with a knowledgeable physician and maintaining as healthy a lifestyle as possible (stopping smoking, for example), your risk of losing your kidneys can drop quite low. While it's difficult to estimate risk precisely, the odds that you will live out your life without losing your kidneys are very good, probably 95% or better.

A Realistic Perspective

So does diabetes pose a potentially serious threat to your health? Of course it does! If you believe that you are not vulnerable to the complications of diabetes or that the risks are so low as to be unimportant, you are wrong. However, if you feel doomed by diabetes, you may be overestimating your actual risks. And you may not be appreciating that your own actions can have an enormous positive impact on reducing those risks. If you are uncertain about what your actual risks are, don't be shy about asking your doctor—the truth can only help you.

Taking action—for example, working to manage blood glucose better—has been shown to stabilize or even improve many long-term complications. Look at the box above to get an idea of your actual risks for developing complications such as blindness and kidney disease.

Just because you have a friend or a relative who developed a terrible complication doesn't mean that the same will happen to you. Diabetes affects each person differently. Also, if you are comparing yourself to someone who struggled with diabetes-related medical problems many years ago ("Twenty years ago, soon after my mom developed diabetes, one of her feet was amputated!"), please remember that your situation is not the same. The past few years have brought tremendous advances in diabetes care that make it easier to achieve and benefit from good diabetes management.

Learning about the Benefits of Good Diabetes Care

For Nora, learning about good care was certainly the most powerful of the four strategies. It is difficult to stay frightened when you begin to regain a sense of control, a sense that your actions truly matter. You are far from powerless. Your efforts to manage your diabetes CAN make an enormous difference. By reminding yourself that there is always something that you can do to confront the bogeyman of complications (be it beginning a regular exercise program, quitting smoking, checking your feet on a regular basis, or finding the right physician), you are taking a vital step toward the harnessing of your fears.

WHAT DO YOU THINK OF YOUR ODDS NOW?

The underlying theme of these four strategies is that your thoughts determine how frightened you become. After reading through the strategies, you may find that your thoughts are already beginning to change. You may already be thinking about your future a little differently. Want to find out? Please complete Worksheet 10.2. It is a copy of the worksheet that you completed several pages ago, but fill it out without looking back at your previous responses.

When you have finished the worksheet, compare your current answers with your previous responses. If you were feeling overly fearless at the beginning of this chapter, your original responses were probably skewed to the extreme left side of the worksheet. Where are they now? *Any* movement toward the right, especially in response to questions 1–3, is probably a sign of progress.

If you began this chapter feeling doomed, your responses on the first worksheet were probably skewed to the right side on questions 1–3 and to the left side on questions 4–6. If your sense of terror has begun to weaken, then your answers on the second worksheet should probably be more to the center or left on questions 1–3 and/or more to the center or right on questions 3–6.

In truth, as your deeply held beliefs move toward reality, it is likely that you will think about your future with a reasonably small amount of fear—enough to persuade you that good health care is necessary and worthwhile, but not enough to make you feel helpless. Take Bonnie and Len, for example. As they learned how their inner beliefs were causing them to feel so frightened and then challenged those beliefs with the true facts about long-term complications, their feelings began to change. Both began to recover from their overwhelming sense of doom and fear. They felt more hopeful about their futures and more powerful as they realized that their actions could strongly influence their future health. And Len, with his new sense of hope, was inspired to take on the task of managing his diabetes as well as possible.

WORKSHEET 10.2: GUESSING ABOUT MY FUTURE AGAIN

Please respond to each question with your best guess. There are no correct answers, so please do not worry about whether your answer is factually accurate. What is most important is to indicate as honestly as possible what you really believe.

A. What would you estimate are the chances that diabetes will:

1. Negatively impact on your long-term health?

___0 (won't happen) ___1/1,000 (might happen) ___1/100 (a fair chance) ___50/50 (pretty likely) ___1/1 (will happen)

2. Cause you to lose your eyesight?

___0 (won't happen) ___1/1,000 (might happen) ___1/100 (a fair chance) ___50/50 (pretty likely) ___1/1 (will happen)

3. Cause you to suffer serious kidney damage and end up on dialysis?

___0 (won't happen) ___1/1,000 (might happen) ___1/100 (a fair chance) ___50/50 (pretty likely) ___1/1 (will happen)

B. To what degree do you think that taking good care of your diabetes could reduce your risk of:

4. Suffering negative consequences to your health over the years?

___It wouldn't help. ___It would help a little. ___It would help a fair amount. ___It would help a great deal.

5. Losing your eyesight?

___It wouldn't help. ___It would help a little. ___It would help a fair amount. ___It would help a great deal.

6. Suffering serious kidney damage and ending up on dialysis?

___It wouldn't help. ___It would help a little. ___It would help a fair amount. ___It would help a great deal.

CHAPTER 11
Depression and Diabetes: A Tough Combination

W e all go through times when the stresses of life become overwhelming, at least temporarily, and we are overcome by a sense of melancholy or gloom. These dark times tend to come and go. They are a natural and understandable part of the human condition. Unfortunately, many people find that such feelings of sadness and despair stay and continue to deepen over time. The sense of gloom can become a constant companion. In these cases, everything is soon affected—ability to think clearly, quality of sleep, family relationships, and more. When this becomes severe, we refer to it as *major depression*. Major depression can have a heavy impact on the quality of life and can even become a life-threatening problem. To make matters even worse, when major depression is combined with diabetes, a terrible interaction often occurs: Depression can make it more difficult to manage diabetes, and in turn, diabetes can make it harder to recognize and treat depression.

In this chapter, we will look at the bad news and the good news about depression and diabetes. The bad news is that depression is common among people with diabetes, is very painful, and has a terrible impact on diabetes self-management. The good news is that almost all forms of depression can be successfully treated. If you've been living under the burden of depression, this does not have to continue!

Let's begin by considering the tales of Henry and Andrea.

HENRY'S STORY

When I first met Henry, he was 32 years old and had been living with type 1 diabetes for 8 years. A bright and charming bachelor, he had been living with his parents since losing his job as a software engineer several years earlier. He had recently found work at a local department store, but this brought him little pleasure. The job was of no interest to him, there was little opportunity for advancement, and he was earning a mere fraction of his former pay. As he described it, "I feel adrift in my life, like a boat on a great ocean. All around me I can see boats passing to and fro, a sense of adventure, romance, and excitement in their wake. But there is no wind in my sails and so I just float here alone, day after day, with ever diminishing hope that anything in my life will ever change or get better." Also, Henry had begun sleeping quite poorly; in fact, he felt tired most of the time and reported that "everything seems like an effort."

Over the past few years, his diabetes management had slipped as well. He continued to take his insulin regularly, but he had not checked his blood glucose in many months. And he had no meal plan at all. He had recently had a glycated hemoglobin (HbA1c) test that indicated his average blood glucose level was well over 300 mg/dl.

Regarding his diabetes, he felt that he was "just going through the motions." He felt hopeless in the face of diabetes, feeling that the disease was going to kill him sometime soon and that there was really nothing he could do about it.

ANDREA'S STORY

For many years, Andrea had lived a satisfying and enjoyable life. Married for more than 40 years, she and her husband had successfully raised three healthy children. In addition, she had completed a long career as a primary school teacher, winning a host of awards, and had retired several years earlier at age 65. After retirement, she had expected that she would have more time for relaxation and that her days would be peaceful and contented. To her surprise, she felt edgy most of the time. Most of her days were spent working aimlessly on household tasks about which she cared little and arguing about serious as well as silly things with her husband.

Over time, Andrea felt more and more grumpy. It was becoming increasingly difficult to get a good night's sleep. She would toss and turn all night and often found herself waking early in the morning and unable to return to sleep. She felt lonely and tired most of the time. She found it tough to concentrate on anything and was slowly losing interest in most of the things that had previously given her pleasure. Without a real job to accomplish, Andrea was feeling more and more worthless. She soon began having frequent thoughts about her own death.

Andrea had been living with type 2 diabetes for more than 10 years and, until recently, had never found it very difficult to manage. Since retirement, she had developed a fondness for late-night snacking, indulging primarily in crackers, cookies, and ice cream. Her blood glucose was now averaging well above 230 mg/dl, and she was gaining weight. Andrea's doctor had recommended that she switch to insulin, but she was not willing to do it. Andrea could tell that things were beginning to fall apart in her life, both physically and emotionally. She knew that she needed to take some positive action, but she didn't know where to start or where she could find the motivation to even begin.

MORE THAN THE BLUES

Unknown to Andrea and Henry, they both had most of the major symptoms that are used to diagnose major depression. These include negative changes in feelings (such as loss of pleasure and sad mood), thoughts (such as feelings of worthlessness and recurrent thoughts of death), and behaviors (such as insomnia, chronic fatigue, and weight gain). Like Andrea and Henry, many people suffer in silence. In some cases, no one recognizes that something is wrong. In others, the person who is suffering never reaches out for help. And without help, the pain of depression may continue year after year.

Andrea and Henry's experiences highlight the fact that depression is much more than just feeling sad. It does not occur because the individual has a "weak mind" or is "crazy." Rather, depression can strike any of us, regardless of how successful, intelligent, or emotionally stable we may be.

Unfortunately, depression is not a rare event. Among the general population, approximately 5% will experience major depression at some time in their lives. However, among those people with diabetes, the rate is *tripled.*

About 15% will experience major depression. It doesn't matter what type of diabetes you have; this dramatically increased risk applies to those with type 1 as well as type 2. Women, especially those in the middle ages of their lives, seem to be at the highest risk of all.

When the milder forms of depression are included, researchers find that 25–30% of people with diabetes are significantly depressed at any one time. Clearly a large number of people with diabetes are likely to encounter depression at least once in their lives. This is especially worrisome because depression can sap your motivation and make it even harder to deal with diabetes self-care tasks.

But how much should you really worry about all this? After all, sad times come and go, just like cloudy days are eventually followed by sunny ones. So what's the big deal? The big deal is that depression is not just a sad mood. Not only is it more powerful and more crippling than sadness, it is like an unwelcome houseguest that doesn't want to leave. Recent studies have evaluated diabetes patients who were treated for major depression (primarily with antidepressant medication) and followed them for 5 years after treatment. Approximately 80% became severely depressed again. The average patient suffered four more bouts with depression, each episode lasting about 14 months. Thus, without powerful intervention, the natural course of depression can be chronic and severe, especially for those with diabetes. The unwelcome houseguest may eventually leave, but it is likely to return.

THE CAUSES OF DEPRESSION

What causes depression? The causes may vary depending on the person, but in most cases it is due to a combination of factors, including

- biology
- social environment
- styles of thinking

We know that biology can play an important role. If you have close relatives who have suffered with depression (especially parents or siblings), then your risk of depression is higher than it would be for other people. Also, a disturbance in a brain or body system may lay the groundwork for depression. For example, depression can occur if there are major changes in your sleep cycle or stress-related hormonal changes. In some cases, even common medications can lead to changes in your brain chemistry that make depression more likely to happen.

Your social environment can also contribute to depression. Job and family stresses, loss of a loved one, and feelings of loneliness all increase the odds that depression will occur.

In addition, there are particular styles of thinking that foster depression. People who typically see themselves as powerless or out of control in their lives are much more likely to become seriously depressed at some point. They have, unfortunately, developed a distorted view of how the world works. It seems that all the bad things in the universe can affect them, but that they are unable to affect the universe. In other words, they come to believe that their own actions just don't matter.

WHAT'S DIABETES GOT TO DO WITH IT?

Diabetes can make depression more likely. For example, when your blood glucose levels are always high, you may feel more down and lethargic. Many people do not know that elevated blood glucose levels can lead to significant changes in mood, including such feelings as melancholy and increased fatigue. For some people, this occurs so gradually that they hardly notice that they are feeling differently. Frequent high and low blood glucose levels can also be quite exhausting, which can help to create the opportunity for depression to appear. In some cases, regaining control of blood glucose levels may cause a substantial improvement in depression.

The ongoing emotional struggle of coping with diabetes can also lead to depression. When you feel that you are constantly failing with your diabetes, when you feel hopeless in the face of long-term complications, when you feel alone with diabetes, these are all feelings that can lead to diabetes burnout and, eventually, depression.

Why are people with diabetes more likely to develop depression? The truth is that anyone who is living with a chronic illness has an increased chance of becoming depressed. But there may be something particularly difficult about diabetes. Diabetes and depression often interact with each other, creating a difficult, downward spiral. For example, both Andrea's and Henry's depression led to a loss of motivation and poorer diabetes self-care (as Henry told me when we first met, "Control my eating? Who cares?!"). In turn, this led to consistently high blood glucose levels, followed by greater fatigue and lethargy. This made their depression worse, leading to a further loss of motivation, and so on. This ongoing vicious cycle can be hard to escape. But the good news is that current treatments for depression are remarkably effective (see below). Almost no one needs to go on this way.

ARE YOU DEPRESSED NOW?

How can you tell if you are depressed? Surprisingly, it is not as easy as you might think. For example, many people experience only the physical symptoms of depression (such as insomnia and appetite changes) without ever really noticing any of the emotional changes. Indeed, in people with diabetes, studies show that depression is recognized and treated in less than one-third of those who are suffering. Less than one-third! The majority of those who have depression never receive any help. They may not even realize what is wrong. Please complete Worksheet 11.1 now to see how *you* are doing.

To determine your total score, you must:

1. Add together all of your responses to questions 1–3, 5–7, 9–11, 13–15, 17–20. This will give you
   TOTAL 1 _____.

2. "Reverse score" your answers to questions 4, 8, 12, and 16. In other words, beginning with question 4, if you circled 0, then give yourself a score of 3. If you circled 1, then your score is 2. If you circled 2, then your score is 1. And if you circled 3, then give yourself a score of 0. Then add together these four new scores. This will give you
   TOTAL 2 _____.

3. Now add together TOTAL 1 and TOTAL 2. This will give your
   TOTAL SCORE _____.

If your total score is 16 or higher, you should consider taking some action right away. Odds are good that you may be suffering with depression, and this may also be affecting your ability to manage your diabetes. The good news is that *depression is often curable*. There is no need for

WORKSHEET 11.1: AM I DEPRESSED?

Please circle the number for each statement that best describes how often you felt or behaved this way DURING THE PAST WEEK:

	Rarely or none of the time (less than 1 day)	Occa- sion- ally or a little of the time (1–2 days)	Some of the time (3–4 days)	All of the time (5–7 days)
1. I was bothered by things that usually don't bother me.	0	1	2	3
2. I did not feel like eating; my appetite was poor.	0	1	2	3
3. I felt that I could not shake off the blues even with help from my family or friends.	0	1	2	3
4. I felt that I was just as good as other people.	0	1	2	3
5. I had trouble keeping my mind on what I was doing.	0	1	2	3
6. I felt depressed.	0	1	2	3
7. I felt that everything I did was an effort.	0	1	2	3
8. I felt hopeful about the future.	0	1	2	3
9. I thought my life had been a failure.	0	1	2	3
10. I felt fearful.	0	1	2	3
11. My sleep was restless.	0	1	2	3
12. I was happy.	0	1	2	3
13. I talked less than usual.	0	1	2	3
14. I felt lonely.	0	1	2	3
15. People were unfriendly.	0	1	2	3
16. I enjoyed life.	0	1	2	3
17. I had crying spells.	0	1	2	3
18. I felt sad.	0	1	2	3
19. I felt that people disliked me.	0	1	2	3
20. I could not get going.	0	1	2	3

suffering to continue when effective treatments are available. If your score is less than 16, it is much less likely that you are living with serious depression. However, you may still be battling with the blues or some milder form of depression. So if you've been feeling down, please read on.

WHAT SHOULD YOU DO?

In the face of depression, what should you do? You should begin by talking to your health care provider. He or she can help you determine what is causing these symptoms. Your health care provider can uncover any physical factors that may be underlying the depression (such as a thyroid disorder or certain prescription medications) and help you develop a plan for treatment. To overcome serious depression, you and your doctor should consider two major strategies: psychotherapy and antidepressant medication.

Psychotherapy

Oddly enough, many people who are significantly depressed avoid psychotherapy. They feel that it is just for people who are "weak," and they believe that they can take care of their problems on their own. On the contrary, those in psychotherapy are the brave ones. They have been willing to risk confrontation with their personal fears and vulnerabilities. And there is good scientific evidence that structured psychotherapy with a mental health professional can help people overcome depression. In particular, a psychotherapy approach that includes *cognitive-behavioral strategies* seems to be effective. Studies show that more than half of those patients who receive such treatment recover from their depression quickly, usually within 3 months.

In this type of action-oriented counseling, the psychotherapist and patient team up to figure out how the patient's thoughts, feelings, and actions may be contributing to the depressive disorder. They then develop specific strategies for making necessary changes. In Andrea's case, for example, her psychotherapist helped her to realize that her depression had been triggered by her retirement, which had led her to the incorrect belief that she was no longer needed and that her life no longer had value. After challenging these negative thoughts and by encouraging new action (Andrea began volunteering at a local elementary school), a cascade of changes soon followed. Andrea's self-esteem began to lift. And this was followed by new energy, an improvement in her sleep, and a closer relationship with her husband. These types of action-oriented psychotherapy approaches are designed to help people cope better with stressful life circumstances and can also be helpful in preventing depression from returning.

Antidepressant Medication

There are three major classes of antidepressant drugs:
- Tricyclic antidepressants. The most well-known is amitryptiline, or Elavil.
- SSRIs (or selective serotonin reuptake inhibitors). The most common one in this class is fluoxetine, better known as Prozac.
- MAO inhibitors (monoamine oxidase inhibitors). These are used least often of the three classes, mostly because they require a special diet.

As with psychotherapy, more than half of the people who receive antidepressant medications recover quickly from their depression.

Despite well-documented benefits, antidepressant drugs have developed a bad reputation over the years. Their use can still lead to people being—or feeling—stigmatized. The truth is that antidepressants are not addictive, and they are not "happy pills." In most cases, they can help people feel more like their old selves. And in combination with psychotherapy, they can help people confront the very real and difficult beliefs, feelings, and situations that need to be resolved. Antidepressants alone are probably the best choice for patients who cannot talk about their problems and for those who don't have the time or money available for psychotherapy.

Nonmedical Strategies

Although reaching out for professional help is the most powerful and important thing that you can do, there are additional steps that you can take on your own to combat depression. Indeed, given that feelings of powerlessness are so closely linked to depression, the mere act of taking ANY positive action is likely to be a valuable step. So consider the following four strategies as well.

1. Exercise. Take action to become physically active, especially if you tend to be a couch potato. A brief walk in the neighborhood each morning (or any time!) is a good way to clear your head and reduce stress (not to mention all the other benefits of physical exercise on diabetes and general health). Also, there is good evidence that regular physical activity may generate biological changes that may aid in reducing depression. So you don't even have to enjoy it. Just walk each day for 1 week, and then decide for yourself whether your mood has improved and whether it was worth doing. (By the way, if starting a regular exercise program like this sounds too overwhelming, please see chapter 8.)

2. Find a confidante. One of the toughest things about major depression is the isolation. Even when you are surrounded by a loving family, it is easy to feel alone and on your own, feeling that no one understands (or can understand) what you are going through. Take a risk by reaching out and making real contact with one person. Ask him or her to listen to you and to talk with you, but not to try to solve your problems. Having a confidante, someone who can really know you, can have a very significant impact on overcoming depression. If a confidante is not possible, put your thoughts and feelings to paper. Specifically, start a journal or write a letter to someone in the world that you trust. You may never share your journal or mail your letter, but there is good evidence that even the act of writing down your thoughts and feelings can have a major influence on your mood.

3. Avoid all attempts at self-medication. Unfortunately, the most common, and most foolish, treatment for depression is the liberal use of alcohol (and/or recreational drugs). Although excessive use of booze can be a temporary escape, taking you away from depression and dulling the pain for a short while, it actually serves over time to *worsen* depression. In the biological arena, for example, excessive alcohol use interferes with the body's ability to enter a state of deep, restful sleep. Thus, frequent boozing leads you to become increasingly deprived of restorative sleep. This results in increasing fatigue as the days pass. If you are suffering with depression and you are drinking excessively, you are pouring gasoline onto a fire. At this stage, seeking outside help is critical.

4. Improve your blood glucose control. As noted earlier, high blood glucose levels can lead to chronic fatigue and other changes in mood that can worsen depression. By bringing blood glucose levels nearer to the normal range, many people find that their moods brighten and their energy levels climb. For example, early in the course of psychotherapy, Henry returned to monitoring his blood glucose regularly, which soon led to a major change in his insulin usage. Within the week, his mood and energy improved. And this provided the push he needed to pursue changes that he had been considering for many months (for example, actively looking for a new, more satisfying job). Thus, as one step toward overcoming depression, you might want to consult with your physician about taking more aggressive action to improve your diabetes management, especially if your blood glucose levels are always high.

In conclusion, if you are suffering with major depression, please know that you are not alone and that there is no need to give up hope. As you have seen here, depression is remarkably common in people with diabetes, and this is partly due to the unfortunate body and mind interaction between diabetes and depression. The good news is that depression is absolutely treatable. By consulting with your health care provider, you can set up an effective treatment plan that may involve psychotherapy, antidepressant medications, and/or a host of personal behavior changes. So don't wait any longer!

CHAPTER 12
What You Don't Know Can't Hurt You (or Can It?): Understanding and Overcoming Denial

Denial. It is a term that is tossed around a lot when people are talking about diabetes, but it is rarely understood. Unfortunately, some health care providers use it to belittle or dismiss their patients. Spouses and other family members often use this expression as well. For example:

■ "Mr. Smith has not done what I have recommended that he do; therefore, he is denying his diabetes."

■ "My wife eats anything she wants to eat, even though she knows that this is having a terrible effect on her blood sugars. Clearly, she is in denial."

In most cases, these types of blanket accusations are unfair, unnecessarily hostile, and inaccurate. An individual might not follow his doctor's recommendation for all sorts of reasons—because he didn't understand what he was being asked to do, because he didn't want to make the suggested change, or because the recommendation was unreasonable. Similarly, many people stray from healthy self-care actions, such as eating well, because of factors that have nothing to do with denial. To be honest, however, there is an important nugget of truth here. The degree to which you ignore the seriousness of diabetes or try to avoid thinking about the illness can play a large role in your overall health for years to come. Denial is a critical problem that must be addressed.

THE ESSENCE OF DENIAL

To what degree is denial a problem for you? In reality, if you were truly in denial of your diabetes, you wouldn't be reading this. This would be the last book in the world that you would choose to pick up! But what about *partial* denial? Do you pay as much attention to your diabetes as you think you should? Do you feel that you have truly accepted diabetes? And to what degree do you need to accept diabetes? To reflect on these issues, consider once again the cases of Mel and Sam, two gentlemen whom you met in chapter 1.

Mel was the 29-year-old carpenter with type 1 diabetes who was infuriated about the illness and tried to think about it as little as possible. He took his insulin each day but had never followed a meal plan, hardly ever checked his blood glucose, and almost never saw a doctor. Sam was the 66-year-old businessman with type 2 diabetes who had seen his father die from diabetes complications and was certain that he would share the same fate. Feeling doomed, he ate anything he wanted, hardly ever exercised, and didn't seem to mind that his blood glucose, blood pressure, and cholesterol were all dangerously out of whack.

What Mel and Sam shared was a common belief about the value of ignoring diabetes. For both of them, living with diabetes was like standing in the path of an oncoming freight train. The train may be far off in the distance and it may be moving slowly, but it is coming. The train cannot be stopped, and there is no way to get off the tracks, so the best thing to do is just pretend it isn't coming. This is the essence of denial.

THE POSITIVE SIDE OF DENIAL

Denial is one particular way of trying to cope with strong, negative feelings about diabetes, especially when everything is feeling out of your control. In fact, if you are struggling with diabetes burnout, denial may look like the best answer. If you are infuriated, frustrated, depressed, guilt-ridden, or frightened about diabetes, then trying to ignore the illness can seem like an almost sensible action to take. Perhaps a better way to understand this remarkable ability is to think of it as *compartmentalization*. You do not really forget you have diabetes (few people are *that* good at denial), but you can manage to put it into another mental compartment. And this is not necessarily a bad thing to do. At times, denying, or compartmentalizing, diabetes can have positive benefits. For example, when diabetes is first diagnosed or when you need a "vacation" from your diabetes.

At First Diagnosis

When you learned that you had diabetes, how did you respond? Like many people, you may have denied the diagnosis at first: "That's impossible! I feel fine." "There is no diabetes in my family; you must be mistaken." "I am certain that your tests must be wrong." In this case, denial was a somewhat healthy and protective response. It helped you to avoid becoming emotionally overwhelmed. Thus, you were able to continue to function at home and at work throughout the next days and weeks, while your brain slowly digested the reality of the diagnosis.

On a Little Vacation

The mental and physical effort that diabetes requires can be exhausting; almost everyone needs a break from time to time. To set themselves free from the pressures, the decisions, and even the memory that they have diabetes, many people have found a way to put diabetes aside for a short while. Perhaps one night a week you dine out and eat anything you want. Or you take an occasional day off from blood glucose monitoring. For that period of time, it can seem that you don't have diabetes. Think of this as "vacationing" from your diabetes, rather than denying it. When you structure these breaks into your life in a *safe* way, they can be good for you. Like a real vacation, they can help you to feel renewed and more inspired to care for your health.

Positive Health Benefits

There may be times when denial has a positive effect on health. At a Connecticut hospital, researchers interviewed 30 men when they were hospitalized for a heart attack or heart surgery. Surprisingly, the men who spent the fewest days in intensive care and recovered the most quickly were those who were the strongest deniers. These were the men who tended to minimize the seriousness of their heart problems. They made such comments as "this is no big deal" or "this won't affect my life very much." By denying, or compartmentalizing, their worries in this manner, these men not only protected themselves from becoming emotionally overwhelmed, but they also were able to positively influence how quickly their bodies mended, at least in the short-term. Could denial have a similarly positive effect on diabetes? Perhaps—but as you will see, there is a serious price to be paid.

THE NEGATIVE CONSEQUENCES OF DENIAL

Although there may be positive benefits to denial, they are—to be truthful—fairly few in number. Usually, the consequences of denial are negative. The critical factor that determines whether denial will be helpful or harmful is *flexibility*. The ability to ignore diabetes, or to ignore anything in your life that is too upsetting or aggravating, is a valuable tool that can help you cope during those difficult times when there is nothing else you can do to resolve the situation. Occasional diabetes "vacations" are necessary.

The problem begins, however, when denial becomes your *only* way of coping with difficult situations. You are no longer flexible about when you use denial as a tool. Instead, it is your way of life. The response to all diabetes aggravations, big and small, becomes "I'm just not going to think about diabetes anymore." Like Mel and Sam, you may end up on permanent vacation from your diabetes. And this means trouble. Study after study have shown that people who use denial as their primary way of coping with diabetes tend to manage their illness more poorly and have high blood glucose levels.

Even in the Connecticut hospital study described above, denial spelled trouble over time. Although those men who minimized the importance of their heart problems recovered more quickly during their hospital stay, they fared much more poorly over the longer term. During the year that followed, they were less likely to make healthy lifestyle changes, and they spent much more time back in the hospital.

ARE YOU IN DENIAL?

How can you tell if you, or someone you know, is ignoring diabetes? Here are some ways of thinking that should serve as warning signs:

"I just have a touch of sugar." If you describe your diabetes in this manner, you may be avoiding the realization that you have a serious illness. To be fair, statements like these are sometimes due to a lack of knowledge rather than denial. However, if you have been diagnosed with diabetes and still choose to think of it as a "touch of sugar," you are making a serious mistake that can harm your health.

"I have borderline diabetes." Claiming that you have borderline diabetes is like claiming that you are borderline pregnant. Either you have diabetes or you don't. Confusion about the role of insulin is often to blame. It is not uncommon to meet people with type 2 diabetes who believe that they are "borderline" because they are not taking insulin. In other words, they believe that diabetes is not real unless you require insulin. And they believe that high blood glucose cannot harm you as long as your diabetes is merely "borderline." These are nice thoughts, but they're wrong!

It's true that sometimes this has nothing to do with denial. In some cases, the health care provider may be responsible for actually putting forward this mysterious diagnosis, a diagnosis that does not exist. In other cases, a personal lack of knowledge is to blame. However, many people manage to combine their lack of knowledge with their need to deny the diagnosis. Thus, after learning that they have diabetes, they *reinterpret* the diagnosis on their own to mean merely "borderline."

"There is no need to check my blood sugar level; it is just going to be high again." If this is a constant refrain, you probably believe there is no need to *ever* check your blood glucose. By avoiding the act of monitoring, you make it easier to pretend that you don't have diabetes. By eluding any feedback about the status of your blood glucose, you can pretend that your high blood glucose levels are not *that* high or that they can't really hurt you. (Please note, however, that a statement like this sometimes has more to do with feeling powerless—"There is nothing I can do about these high blood sugar readings!"—than with denial.)

"Diabetes is no big deal." Want to bet? As in the previous examples, this statement may sometimes result from being poorly informed rather than from being in denial. However, if you have learned about the seriousness of diabetes and have chosen to ignore or forget that fact, then you are committing a grave disservice to yourself.

"Why bother taking care of my diabetes? No matter what you do, everybody dies eventually!" On the surface, this sounds like a convincing argument for ignoring your diabetes care. There is nothing you can do to avoid your eventual death (nothing can stop the oncoming freight train), so why make the effort to stop smoking, lower your blood glucose, or begin an exercise program? If you, like Sam, allow this line of reasoning to determine how you manage (or don't manage) your diabetes, you are making a serious error in logic. Good health care is likely to extend your life and, perhaps even more importantly, to extend your years of life as an independent, healthy person. You should bother taking care of your diabetes because it will have an enormous positive impact on the quality of your life, regardless of the number of years that you have remaining on this planet.

WHY DENY?

If you tend to minimize or ignore diabetes, then it is likely that you are awash with unpleasant feelings about the disease—feelings that you cannot control and would rather not think about. But there are three other factors that may play a role in denial:

- Belief in the power of magical thinking. Ignoring diabetes becomes even more attractive when you start to think that denial has magical properties—to believe "what I don't know or don't think about can't hurt me." You may believe that by thinking about diabetes as little as possible you are somehow protecting your body from all the terrible things that poorly controlled diabetes might do. But of course high blood sugar is there whether you check it or not, and it will do damage whether you think about it or not.

- Refusal to surrender. Like Mel, there are many people who view diabetes as an ongoing battle for personal independence. They are preoccupied with the concern that "either diabetes will control my life or I will." Compromise is not possible. For people who refuse to surrender, making the effort to manage their diabetes means losing control over their daily lives.

They believe that accepting diabetes signifies defeat. So ignoring diabetes becomes a way to avoid losing the battle.

▌ Not knowing any better. If your ideas about diabetes, especially type 2 diabetes, are gathered from the experiences and convictions of loved ones (whose beliefs may be seriously outdated) or a physician who is not knowledgeable about diabetes, you may not realize how serious diabetes is. If you have somehow come to believe that diabetes cannot cause you any serious harm, it is understandable that you might choose to ignore it.

OVERCOMING DENIAL

To begin, please realize that denial of diabetes is based on the false idea that there is nothing you can do to improve your situation. Ignoring something bad that is happening to you makes perfect sense *only if there really is nothing you can do about it*. If that freight train actually is bearing down on you and there is no way to stop or avoid it, then some form of denial will help you to pass your last few minutes peacefully. In that case, denial is a smart choice. But this is not the case with diabetes. The freight train may be coming, but you are not tied to those tracks. You are not powerless. No matter how angry, frightened, saddened, or overwhelmed by diabetes you are, you can take action to improve your health.

Overcoming denial means having the courage to open your eyes, look around at your situation, and move! Here are five strategies that can help you to do just that.

1. Make room in your life for unpleasant feelings about diabetes. Chronic denial is most likely to occur when you have no other way to deal with your feelings

FIVE STRATEGIES FOR OVERCOMING DENIAL

1. Make room in your life for unpleasant feelings about diabetes.
2. Learn about the hidden beliefs concerning diabetes that are causing you to feel so miserable.
3. Challenge the beliefs that are driving you crazy.
4. Let your hair down with a friend.
5. Get regular feedback about your own health status.

about diabetes. Bottling up your emotions seems like the only solution. But it is usually a lousy solution. It is important to recognize that all of your feelings about diabetes are understandable and probably quite normal. Almost everyone goes through times when diabetes makes them feel aggravated, depressed, terrified, wracked with guilt, infuriated, boxed in, worried, and much more. It has happened before, and it will happen again. Corny as it may sound, the first step in overcoming such misery is to take a good look at your innermost feelings about diabetes.

Take Sam, for example. His doctor as well as everyone in the family had tried to convince Sam to take better care of his diabetes. All to no avail. As it turned out, what Sam needed—even to his surprise—was to talk about his dad. In one of our most important sessions, Sam told me the haunting story of his father's death. Beginning with a simple foot infection, Sam's father had been overwhelmed by diabetes-related complications in a few months. The loss of his left leg was soon followed by severe vision loss due to retinopathy and then the development of serious kidney damage. This proud, strong man was soon reduced to an invalid, and his spirit had been crushed. His death soon after seemed a blessing.

Sam had never discussed or really even allowed himself to think about how horrified he had been at what happened to his father. Now that he was letting himself examine and reexperience these old memories, Sam realized how truly frightened about diabetes he was. Oddly enough, by allowing himself to confront his true feelings, Sam could begin to gain some perspective on them. His father's experience had taught Sam that diabetes was a killer, but this doesn't have to be true—especially with current medical technology. With his feelings no longer blocking his ability to think clearly, Sam could understand that he did not have to share his father's fate, that good care could help him live a long and healthy life.

One of the most important lessons to learn from Sam's story is that unpleasant feelings like these don't go away when you ignore them. Instead, they hover nearby and freeze you into emotional immobility: you cannot really be free of these feelings until you do something about them. By allowing yourself to go ahead and feel and examine your own feelings, you begin to transform them. And as your thinking begins to clear, these feelings can lead you into health-promoting action rather than continued paralysis. For another illustration of how helpful this strategy can be, see what happened to Mel in chapter 7.

It is easy to think, "I just don't like diabetes and that's that." In most cases, it is more difficult to look deeply into the swamp of your own emotional state. Take a few moments now to complete Worksheet 12.1 and consider how you really feel about diabetes.

WORKSHEET 12.1: YOUR EMOTIONAL STRUGGLE WITH DIABETES

A. Listed below are some of the difficult emotions people experience in their day-to-day struggle with diabetes. Think about the degree to which each of these feelings may be present in you, especially as you think about living with diabetes, and circle the appropriate number.

	Not at all		Somewhat		Very much	
1. Angry	1	2	3	4	5	6
2. Sad	1	2	3	4	5	6
3. Frightened	1	2	3	4	5	6
4. Anxious	1	2	3	4	5	6
5. Guilty	1	2	3	4	5	6
6. Frustrated	1	2	3	4	5	6
7. Hopeless	1	2	3	4	5	6
8. Lonely	1	2	3	4	5	6
9. Ashamed	1	2	3	4	5	6
10. Defeated	1	2	3	4	5	6

B. Giving special attention to those emotions that you scored the highest, please describe how you feel about diabetes. What is living with this illness like for you? Record your feelings here as clearly and honestly as you can, as if you were writing a brief letter to someone close to you:

_____

_____

_____

_____

_____

_____

_____

_____

2. Learn about the hidden beliefs concerning diabetes that are causing you to feel so miserable. This is the same peculiar idea that we addressed in chapter 10—the notion that your beliefs about diabetes can strongly influence your emotional state. By exposing these hidden beliefs (often quite old and irrational) to the light of your conscious mind, you can begin to decide whether or not to keep them, change them, or toss them out. In other words, your job is to identify and challenge those important inner "truths," which—you may discover—may not be so true after all.

▪ **"I must take care of my diabetes *perfectly.*"** If lurking behind your difficulty with accepting diabetes is the fact that you are infuriated with the illness, feel boxed in by the overwhelming demands, or despair that you can never manage diabetes successfully, perhaps the belief that you need to be perfect is the real culprit. The solution to the problem of denial may be to challenge this unreasonable belief and to establish more sensible expectations for your diabetes care. (See chapters 9 and 18 for more.)

▪ **"Nothing I do can stop diabetes complications."** If you feel helpless or hopeless about diabetes, terrified about the future, or furious about the seemingly pointless demands of good self-care, perhaps these feelings are being fueled by the underlying belief that complications are unstoppable. While this belief is widespread, it is—fortunately—wrong. For more details and solutions to this problem, see chapter 10.

▪ **"My personal needs must always be secondary to the needs of my diabetes."** Many people imagine that they must be slaves to their diabetes. Few are willing or able to tolerate this imagined relationship,

A NOTE FOR FRIENDS AND FAMILY: HELPING THE PERSON WHO DOESN'T WANT TO BE HELPED

So you think your loved one is not taking good enough care of his diabetes. You want to help, but your help is not appreciated. You should probably back off and leave him alone, but it is difficult to watch someone you care about hurt himself. You feel like a nag if you try to help, but you feel irresponsible if you don't try to help. What a terrible bind! Here are some DOs and DON'Ts for overcoming this problem:

1. **DON'T assume that you know what your loved one is really thinking or feeling.** It is easy to say someone is in denial about diabetes, but an explanation like this is almost always inadequate. Human beings are terrible at mind reading! You can't know what anyone is thinking or feeling unless you ask.

2. **DO try and understand how your loved one's actions make sense from *his* perspective.** Ask him about his feelings about diabetes and concerns about the future. Try to understand diabetes from his point of view, without interrupting him and without judging him. The only way you can ever really understand why your loved one seems not to be taking care of his diabetes is to ask him directly.

3. **DON'T offer advice unless you're asked for it.** You may already know that offering advice without being asked is not very helpful, but it can be tempting to make suggestions ("You really need to start checking your blood sugars") even when you know the response is not going to be a good one. Don't do it!

4. **DO offer to help.** During a quiet time when neither of you is angry or upset, let your loved one know that you are concerned about his health and that you would like to help. Let him know that you don't want to be a nag, but you don't know how else to aid him. Ask what you can do, if anything, to be of assistance. Emphasize your understanding that he must be in control of any diabetes-related help that is offered or taken.

A NOTE FOR FRIENDS AND FAMILY: HELPING THE PERSON WHO DOESN'T WANT TO BE HELPED *(continued)*

5. **DO remind him on a regular basis that you love him.** Sometimes there is nothing that you can do about your loved one's diabetes-related actions (or lack of actions), so you must quietly back off. While respecting his wishes, you can find ways to remind him that you care about him, that you are always rooting for him, and that you are on his side. By building a caring alliance with your loved one, you make positive change in the future more likely.

6. **DO get educated.** In many cases, your loved one will benefit from greater knowledge about diabetes—and you will too. Find the best diabetes education program in your area and enroll in it. You, not him. And if your loved one wants to go with you, *that would be just fine.* Besides being an excellent source of information about diabetes, a good program is a great way to meet others and see how they are coping with similar frustrations.

and so the revolt begins. If you are feeling angry and deprived about diabetes, maybe it is because you have subscribed to this inaccurate belief.

▌ **"Any odd blood sugar reading is a sign that I have done something wrong (or 'bad')."** When you discover that your blood sugar is higher than you expected, do you tend to blame yourself? Or, worse yet, do you feel that your meter is blaming you? If so, you probably believe that you are usually responsible for such fluctuations. And the frustration may make you want to turn your back on your diabetes. But is this underlying belief reasonable and accurate? Although sometimes such blame may be deserved ("Well, I did just eat a huge bag of jelly beans"), there will be many occasions when it is not. For example, after criticizing himself for many months, one of my patients finally realized that his high blood glucose levels were due to an inadequate insulin dosage. Once he was able to directly address this problem with his physician, his high blood glucose all but disappeared. For further discussion of this topic, see chapters 7 and 18.

As you can see, the beliefs that cause trouble are the ones that focus on the absolute: diabetes must be managed *perfectly*, you can *never* slow or stop the development of long-term complications, your personal needs must *always* be secondary to diabetes. No wonder beliefs like these lead only to frustration, anger, fear, and burnout! By looking behind your feelings about diabetes, to the hidden beliefs that are contributing to these difficult emotions, you are taking an important step toward understanding the reasons for ignoring diabetes. And you are preparing for change. To drive this process along, please complete Worksheet 12.2 now.

With this worksheet completed, you may now have acquired a clearer understanding of the unique feelings and beliefs that can cause you to turn your back on diabetes. With these insights, it is now time for action.

3. Challenge the beliefs that are driving you crazy. The beliefs about diabetes that are causing you so much distress may well be in error. But if you have thought this way for many years, it may be hard to consider the possibility of surrendering these beliefs—even if you would like to! At the least, please be willing to question your own deeply held opinions. And remember that just shining the light of consciousness on your old, musty beliefs may help you realize that change is necessary. You might even realize that you need to update the way you think about diabetes.

WORKSHEET 12.2: IDENTIFYING YOUR HIDDEN BELIEFS ABOUT DIABETES

A. Which of the following beliefs, if any, may be contributing to your emotional distress about diabetes? As honestly as you can, please consider the degree to which you agree or disagree with the following statements, then circle the appropriate number. You may have other attitudes that are not listed here. Space is provided for you to record those as well.

	Strongly disagree				Strongly agree	
1. I should take care of my diabetes perfectly.	1	2	3	4	5	6
2. Nothing I do can stop the juggernaut of diabetes complications.	1	2	3	4	5	6
3. My personal needs must always be secondary to the needs of my diabetes.	1	2	3	4	5	6
4. Any high or low blood sugar reading means I have done something wrong (or "bad").	1	2	3	4	5	6
5. Diabetes is not a serious disease.	1	2	3	4	5	6
6. Diabetes cannot harm me.	1	2	3	4	5	6
7. If I don't think about my diabetes, it can't hurt me.	1	2	3	4	5	6
8. Taking good care of my diabetes means that it will control my life.	1	2	3	4	5	6
9. Other_____	1	2	3	4	5	6
10. Other_____	1	2	3	4	5	6

B. As you examine your highest-scoring beliefs, can you see how these attitudes may contribute to the emotional stress factors that you indicated on Worksheet 12.1? Selecting the one or two beliefs that you agreed with most strongly, please describe how you think these beliefs may have contributed to your difficult feelings about diabetes. As in the previous worksheet, record your thoughts here as

(continued)

What You Don't Know Can't Hurt You (or Can It?)

clearly and honestly as you can, as if you were writing a brief letter to someone close to you:

_____

_____

_____

_____

_____

_____

_____

Please complete the exercise in Worksheet 12.3 to start challenging your beliefs.

Many people find it difficult to challenge their beliefs without convincing information. For example, perhaps you find it difficult to believe that good diabetes care really can slow or halt the development of complications. In that case, what you need is additional knowledge. By enrolling in a diabetes education group, attending a local support group, or questioning your doctor, you can get the additional answers that you need. Becoming knowledgeable about diabetes can dramatically transform even the most destructive of beliefs, replacing hopelessness with hope, vagueness with clarity, and confusion with confidence.

4. Let your hair down with a friend. Making the effort to confront your own mixed bag of subconscious feelings and beliefs about diabetes is usually too difficult to do on your own. You need to find someone with whom you can share and think through these innermost thoughts. Confiding in someone you can trust can help you to get the

WORKSHEET 12.3: CHALLENGING YOUR BELIEFS ABOUT DIABETES

A. Please examine the following list of flawed beliefs (from Worksheet 12.2) and note the corresponding factual statements to the right of each belief. Please give special attention to those with which you agreed (scoring 4 or higher on Worksheet 12.2). If you listed additional attitudes on Worksheet 12.2, you may wish to list them here and consider what the more accurate statements might be. Space is provided below for this purpose.

1. I should take care of my diabetes perfectly.

   1. I should take care of my diabetes as well as I can, with the understanding that no one can do it perfectly.

2. Nothing I do can stop diabetes complications.

   2. Managing my diabetes well will dramatically reduce my risk of developing complications.

3. My personal needs must always be secondary to the needs of my diabetes.

   3. Working with my health care team, I can find ways to take care of my diabetes and, at the same time, have a life!

4. Any high or low blood sugar reading means I have done something wrong (or "bad").

   4. High and low blood sugars can occur for reasons that have nothing to do with my actions.

5. Diabetes is not a serious disease.

   5. Diabetes is a very serious disease.

6. Diabetes cannot harm me.

   6. Without proper care, diabetes will harm me.

7. If I don't think about my diabetes, it can't hurt me.

   7. Poorly controlled diabetes can hurt me whether I am thinking about it or not.

8. Taking good care of my diabetes means that diabetes will control my life.

   8. Taking good care of my diabetes will require time and effort, but it will allow me to feel more in control of my life.

(continued)

WORKSHEET 12.3: CHALLENGING YOUR BELIEFS ABOUT DIABETES *(continued)*

9. Other _____ 9. Other _____

10. Other _____ 10. Other _____

B. Selecting the one or two beliefs that you agreed with most
   strongly in Worksheet 12.2, please describe how you might
   be able to use the corresponding factual statements to
   begin challenging your beliefs.

_____

_____

_____

_____

_____

_____

_____

support and perspective that is so necessary for making
sense out of your own emotions and attitudes. You might
choose a close friend or family member, attend a diabetes
support group, or like Mel and Sam, you might elect to talk
with a diabetes-knowledgeable counselor or therapist.
Sound too difficult? For tips on how to establish these types
of contacts or relationships, see chapter 13.

5. Get regular feedback about your own health status.
It is hard to ignore diabetes and diabetes care when you are
committed to staying informed about the circumstances
of your own health. See a diabetes-knowledgeable physician
on a regular basis and have all of the major, American
Diabetes Association–recommended medical tests
completed (glycated hemoglobin, microalbumin, and
lipid panel) and your blood pressure checked. You should
know the results of these tests and what the results mean.

In all cases, regular blood glucose monitoring will give you information you need as well. Becoming aware of your own health status is a freeing, empowering experience that is an important first step toward living a longer and healthier life. Once you realize this, you will find yourself becoming less and less interested in turning your back on diabetes.

Friends, Family, and Health Care Providers

CHAPTER 13
The Secret of the Smoking Room

Ｉt was the oddest thing. Many years ago, when I was a senior psychologist at the Joslin Diabetes Center in Boston, I had the pleasure of working with patients in Joslin's well-known Diabetes Treatment Unit (DTU). The DTU was a wonderful place. Patients from all over the U.S. and all over the world would come to the DTU. They would typically stay for 1 or 2 weeks to participate in classes and receive intensive diabetes care. There was always a wild mix of people, including young and old, rich and poor, foreign and local dignitaries, those who were new to diabetes and those who had been living with it for many decades. Some would come because they were in crisis, others merely for an annual "tune-up." At the end of their stay, I would often ask patients what they most enjoyed about the DTU, what they felt had truly made a difference in their lives. Was it the knowledgeable physicians? The highly competent and caring nursing staff? The informative classes? "The doctors, nurses, other members of the staff, and the classes were all terrific," many told me, "but the most valuable part of the DTU was the smoking room."

The smoking room? How could that be? The smoking room was a small, windowless cubicle where anyone in the DTU who wanted to smoke was exiled (this was, of course, back in the days before smoking was forbidden in most hospitals). It was a grubby, horrible place—even the smokers thought so. The smoke and stale tobacco smells were often so heavy that breathing was almost impossible. And the walls were stained yellow from the ever present clouds of tobacco smoke. Even stranger was that many of the patients who claimed to love the smoking room didn't even smoke! My mission was clear: I needed to uncover the secret of the smoking room.

I began to interview patients in more detail and, against my better judgment, started to spend time in the smoking room. In a few weeks, I had my answer. Patients felt that the smoking room made a big difference in their lives because this was the place where they could hang out and talk with each other. In the smoking room, you could realize that you were not alone, that others shared the same worries, fears, aggravations, and problems that you had. In the smoking room, you could make new friends, learn the very best tips about diabetes management, or gossip about that new DTU physician. For many of these people, even those who had caring and supportive families, this was the first place where they could talk about diabetes honestly and truly be understood. The secret of the smoking room was straightforward: Feeling connected to others, feeling that someone else grasps what living with diabetes is really like for you, feeling that someone cares can make a huge and crucial difference in your diabetes care.

YOUR PERSONAL CHEERLEADER

Over the past decade, numerous research studies have supported this observation. People with the best family support tend to manage their diabetes better and feel better about living with diabetes. The bottom line is that it helps to have someone rooting for you, especially when you are dealing with a trying illness like diabetes. And your personal cheerleader doesn't have to be someone else with diabetes; it can be anybody who has the capacity for understanding and support. A caring friend can help you feel less overwhelmed, can remind you to take your medications, can join you in your exercise program, or can laugh with you about the craziness of diabetes.

I remember one young woman who had been closely managing her diabetes for years. How had she kept up her oomph all this time? "Every morning," she told me, "my husband sits with me at the breakfast table while I check my blood sugars. He congratulates me when the result is in my target range, he worries with me when it's too high, and always we laugh. It's enough to keep me going all day, just knowing that he loves me and cares enough to sit with me and worry with me."

ALONE WITH DIABETES

Of course, the problem is that there aren't too many smoking rooms left out there. Too many people with diabetes feel that they are struggling alone. If you are worried about a lack of support, you are not the only one. My colleagues and I have found that among our patients, about one in three feels isolated with diabetes, that there is no one to whom they can really talk about their feelings about diabetes. Almost the same number feel unsupported, that they aren't getting as much help from family and friends as they need—or want—to take care of their diabetes. And even more feel unappreciated, that friends and family don't really understand how difficult living with diabetes can be.

They may sense a lack of *emotional* support ("No one in my life seems to understand or care") or a lack of *tangible* support ("No one in my life seems willing to take any action to support my diabetes efforts"). Of these people, some experience a lack of support when they feel that their friends or family are not backing them in their diabetes struggle. Others feel unsupported because they don't have any friends or family who are a part of their everyday life. They have little diabetes support because they don't have any emotional support in their lives at all. Consider the example of Ray.

When I first met Ray, he was 61 years old and working as a teacher. A friendly and charming man, he had been divorced for many years and lived alone. Ray had been diagnosed with type 2 diabetes 7 years earlier and had never been able to manage it successfully. He was significantly overweight, and his blood glucose levels ranged between 200 and 300 mg/dl. On numerous occasions, he had set his mind to beginning an exercise program, a new meal plan, or a scheme to check his blood glucose regularly. However, none of Ray's plans ever lasted very long. He would soon return to his old habits.

Ray had a few close friends, but he didn't see them often. And he almost never talked to them about his health problems. Given how poorly he was managing his diabetes, it was just too embarrassing to discuss with anyone. One day, Ray heard me give a talk about the problems of the "diabetes police" (see chapter 14). "A diabetes policeman," he said wistfully, "I'd do almost anything to have one in my life."

Ray was a lonely, isolated fellow, although he certainly didn't want to be. And his need for a diabetes policeman was understandable. What he was really saying was that he wanted a caring someone in his life who would prod him to stay on track with his diabetes management. Like many people, Ray found that it was too difficult for him to make the necessary, long-term lifestyle changes that diabetes demanded without having someone in his life to support him and to ground his efforts—to share healthy meals with him, to care about his blood glucose results, to drive with him to the doctor when he wasn't feeling well, to let him know that he was loved and that his continuing good health mattered. Was this a sign of weakness in Ray's character? Not at all. I would wager that many people find themselves having similar problems.

FRUSTRATIONS WITH YOUR LOVED ONES

Some people may experience a lack of diabetes support even if they are living with family and have plenty of friends. Do any of the following sound familiar to you?

▌ Your loved ones just don't seem to understand why you sometimes get aggravated or frightened about diabetes.

▌ They don't see the need to start buying diet soda or to change the way the rest of the family eats.

▌ They get angry with you for not having more willpower.

▌ They think that diabetes is not that hard to handle and that you should just make more of an effort.

■ They tempt you to join them in eating unhealthy foods. After all, what's the big deal? You look fine.

In any of these cases, opportunities for frustration and misery on all sides abound. Why do such problems develop? Here are the top five reasons.

1. Your family and friends may be uneducated about diabetes. Even though they care about you, your family and friends may not understand that diabetes is a serious disease that requires a fair amount of lifestyle change. They may not understand how tough and frustrating diabetes can be. And they may not realize that making these kinds of difficult behavioral changes in how you eat, exercise, and schedule your activities may require the help and cooperation of everyone. Successful diabetes care demands, in most cases, a family effort.

2. They want to help, but they have developed some odd ideas about how to do so. Friends and family often make the mistake of *mind reading*, of presuming that they know what you are thinking and feeling without having to ask you. So they may decide that you have been too strict with your diabetes self-care and that you need to loosen up ("C'mon, one little bite isn't going to hurt you"). Or they may conclude that you have been too lax and that what you desperately need is some advice ("Y'know, you really should stop eating cookies at night"). When your friends and family never ask you directly about what kind of help you might want, it may be hard to recognize that their peculiar actions are, in fact, attempts at being supportive. Even though their hearts may be in the right place, it is understandable that you might feel alone with your diabetes.

3. They may not see the need to change their own habits or lifestyle. If you are trying to adopt a healthier eating style or become more physically active, your odds of succeeding will be much better if your loved ones join you in making these healthy changes (especially if they live with you). For example, perhaps you've decided that eating lower-fat foods and more vegetables at dinner should be a priority. However, your spouse and children may be perfectly happy with their high-fat, vegetable-free meals. They may understand that you have diabetes and would benefit from these changes, but they do not see why they should be inconvenienced. After all, they don't have diabetes!

4. There may be serious conflict in your family. This is a tough one. If there is a lot of fighting or bad feelings in your family, then it is unlikely you'll feel supported about your diabetes care—or anything. In some cases, disagreements about diabetes are merely the tip of a much larger iceberg, pointing to a much larger breakdown in family relationships.

5. You may never have asked directly for help. Perhaps you feel unsupported because you have never explained to your loved ones how they could help you. Your needs are unique, and there is no way that family and friends can know if you don't tell them. Sometimes, people stubbornly think, "If they really cared about me, they would figure out how to support my efforts." But that's just not fair.

GATHERING THE SUPPORT YOU NEED

There is no doubt that the stresses of living with diabetes are much more likely to wear you down when you don't have someone in your life who is rooting for you, who cares about your welfare. So what to do? To succeed with your diabetes, how can you gain the support that you need? Consider the following four strategies:

> **FOUR STRATEGIES FOR GETTING THE SUPPORT YOU NEED**
>
> 1. Use the subtle approach to enhancing support from your family and friends: Help them get more information about the ins and outs of diabetes.
> 2. Use the not-so-subtle approach to enhancing support from your family and friends: Ask for it!
> 3. Seek out support if you don't have any.
>   - Attend a diabetes support group.
>   - Establish some new friendships.
>   - If your family has been engulfed in conflict for some time, seek professional assistance.
> 4. Examine your own behavior.

1. Use the subtle approach to enhancing support from your family and friends. If your loved ones just don't understand about diabetes, then helping them to become better informed may produce positive changes. You might begin by asking your friends and family whether they might be interested in learning a little more. You could explain what diabetes means, show them how blood glucose monitoring works, and clear up any misunderstandings they may have. You could share relevant published materials with them, such as this book or the American Diabetes Association magazine *Diabetes Forecast*.

Explain the personal side of diabetes to help them understand how this difficult illness has affected your life. Another good option is to invite them to attend a diabetes education program or support group with you. If your family is resistant to joining with you in making some of the healthy eating or activity changes that you are trying to make ("Not go to McDonald's this week? You've got to be joking!"), you could remind them that such changes will benefit them as well—reducing their risk of heart disease, cancer, and more, while positively influencing weight, energy level, and personal well-being.

I have seen many of my patients take these courageous steps with their loved ones. It is remarkable how many family and friends who had been uninvolved and uninterested in diabetes were truly shocked, and fascinated, by the complexities of diabetes and diabetes care. Realizing that diabetes was in fact a bigger deal than they had thought and that their help was needed, they changed their outlook and became more willing to be of aid. Thus, by helping your family and friends learn more about diabetes, you are—unbeknownst to them—involving them. With their new knowledge and understanding, they are more likely to be willing and interested in supporting your self-care efforts.

2. Use the not-so-subtle approach to enhancing support from your family and friends. One of the most effective ways to get the help that you need is to ask for it. This is especially critical if you have been quietly waiting for your loved ones to somehow figure out what you need. No more of that; it's time for you to take action.

As a first step, make a list of some of the ways your family or friends could better support your self-care efforts. Why? Because if you are not clear about the type of help you need, it is unlikely that things can get any better. Let your thoughts run free, and think about what would really help you. As you make your list, avoid the more vague, grand desires ("I think everyone in my family should love me unconditionally"). Try to be as specific as possible and focus on issues relevant to diabetes. Ask yourself the following questions:

- What type of *tangible* support would you like? Someone to exercise with you? Your family deciding to join you in a healthier approach to eating? Someone who would sit with you while you check your blood glucose? A loved one who would go to the doctor with you?
- What type of *emotional* support would you like? A friend who would really try to listen and understand your worries about diabetes? Someone who would congratulate you on all your hard work? A companion who could laugh with you about the absurdities of diabetes?

When you are definite about what you want, it becomes much easier to reach out for help. Select things that are meaningful to you, and remember that you can start with small needs. It is remarkable that sometimes even very small changes can be of enormous value. I remember one young woman, Deirdre, who hated blood glucose monitoring so much, especially in the morning, that she had stopped doing it several years before. When I asked her to complete this exercise, she realized that she simply wanted someone to sit with her each morning while she checked her blood glucose. Luckily, Deirdre had a new housemate whom she could ask. This worked out very successfully. It helped her to monitor more frequently and to feel more at ease with her diabetes. As a bonus, she was delighted to make a new friend.

So what are three or four specific ways in which your loved ones could better support your self-care efforts? Take a moment to write your answers down.

_____

_____

_____

_____

_____

_____

_____

_____

_____

_____

_____

_____

_____

_____

As a second step, select one of the things you wrote, preferably not the most difficult one, and think of someone in your life who you think might be most willing and able to help. Perhaps you are planning to start a walking program and are thinking about asking your neighbor to join you. Perhaps you are trying to reduce high-fat foods in your household and would like your spouse to stop buying all those delicious peanuts. As in these examples, be very specific about how you think this person might be able to support you and your self-care efforts. Consider how you might approach this person. Can you talk about your needs without being hostile or upset? If you are calm and clear, you stand a good chance of establishing the new kind of relationships that will benefit the both of you.

The best way to prepare for this conversation is to rehearse it. Take a few moments now to write a brief letter to the person you have selected, explaining exactly what you need. Remember to include your own thoughts and feelings, including why their help is so important to you. No one has to ever see this letter; you can rip it up and burn it when you are done. The point is simply to practice what you want to say. You will be surprised how something as simple as this will mobilize you for taking action.

Dear _____:

_____

_____

_____

_____

_____

_____

_____

_____

_____

_____

Finally, now that you've thought about how your loved ones might better support you and have selected the first person to approach, do it!

3. Seek out support if you don't have any. The first two strategies presume that you have family and friends who care about you and that you can build on that love and support to get the diabetes-related help that you need. But what if you live alone and feel more isolated than you ever wanted to be? Or you might be living with your family, but there is so much conflict and hostility that you are feeling as lonely, or lonelier, than Ray. Here are three actions to consider:

▌ Attend a diabetes support group. Remember the smoking room? The people who can best understand and aid you in your diabetes struggles may be those who are going through the same thing. Call your local ADA office or local hospital to locate a support group close to you. Commit to attending a single meeting. Don't forget that there are numerous diabetes groups and "electronic communities" on the Internet, providing the opportunity for meeting others and getting emotional support. For many people, these different types of groups serve as a fulfilling way of getting the special support and encouragement that everyone needs.

- Establish some new friendships. Commit yourself to taking some immediate action that will move you in this direction, such as asking a colleague out to lunch, saying hello to one of your neighbors, or joining an organization or social club so that you will have more opportunities to meet new people. Don't be shy; remember that almost everyone else is interested in making new friends too.

- If your family has been engulfed in conflict for some time, seek professional assistance. Perhaps you and your spouse have been barely on speaking terms for years. Perhaps the bad feelings between you and your siblings have poisoned the atmosphere of every family gathering for as long as you can remember. The pressure of ongoing family conflict can be very heavy, making it even more difficult to care about your diabetes. And, let's face it, problems like these can be too difficult to solve on your own. In tough situations like these, ask your health care provider about referral to a mental health professional who is knowledgeable about family therapy. What do you have to lose?

4. Examine your own behavior. Don't forget to consider how your own attitudes and actions may be contributing to your lack of support. If you have been sullenly waiting for your loved ones to figure out that you needed their help, the person who needs to change is you! To be specific, see strategy 2. However, perhaps you have already approached a friend or family member and have been rebuffed. Before blaming them for being selfish, investigate your own role in this drama.

In your approach to your loved ones, were you gruff, aggressive, uncompromising, overly demanding, or inconsiderate of their needs and desires? Do you acknowledge and thank them when they do attempt to help out? For instance, just because you would like your family to stop buying gallons of ice cream so that you won't be faced with that temptation every night, why should they automatically bow to your wishes? Though they may want to help, your loved ones have their own needs and feelings. Any household change that is made should be a sensitive and caring compromise, where everyone's needs are considered. So be cautious as you reach out for support, being aware that your approach may be leading you to frustration. And remember that one of the best ways to overcome problems like these is to try to be as sensitive to your loved one's point of view as your are to your own.

OPENING COMMUNICATION CHANNELS

In the craziness of our daily lives, even a single friend or the smallest gesture of support can have a huge positive impact. Good support can make the difference between long-term success and failure with your diabetes care.

In Ray's case, he finally decided to take the plunge by attending a diabetes support group. He feared that he was going to be faced with a room full of complainers or little old ladies, but he was pleasantly surprised. He enjoyed the group (which he decided to keep attending) and met a nice fellow very much like him who happened to live nearby. They soon decided to join a local health club and to begin exercising together. This was the beginning of Ray's turnaround. Along with other self-care changes, Ray's blood glucose began to improve, and he gained a sense of confidence that he could control his health and his diabetes. And, like Dierdre, he discovered that it was awfully nice to have a new friend.

For those of you who already have family and friends, remember that your loved ones probably have the best of intentions. In most cases, they want to help, but they may not be certain how to do it. And they may be just as frustrated with you as you may be with them. Your job is to open up the channels of communication, providing your loved ones with an opportunity to learn more about diabetes, letting them know about your unique needs in an assertive and sensitive manner, and listening to their concerns and aggravations as well. As you struggle with the everyday problems of diabetes, wouldn't it be nice to have people in your life who are supporting you and rooting for you? The smoking room may be gone, but you can capture the feel of it (hopefully not the smell of it) in your own life.

CHAPTER 14
The Diabetes Police

They come in all shapes and sizes: husbands, wives, parents, children, brothers, sisters, friends, neighbors, coworkers, doctors, nurses, and even complete strangers. They are everywhere. Many of them look so innocent that you'd never suspect anything, until it's too late. As you sleep, they make their secret plans, plotting how to keep you under constant observation and make sure that you stay on the straight and narrow. Why would they do so? Because they are card-carrying members of that secret conspiracy, the "diabetes police."

The diabetes police? Yes, you know who we are talking about. These are your friends, colleagues, and family members who care about you so much that they are going to help you manage your diabetes, *WHETHER YOU LIKE IT OR NOT!* They may treat you like a competent human being in all other ways, but when it comes to diabetes, you are viewed as irresponsible, uneducated, or—worst of all—a diabetes criminal. If you had a slice of cake last night, the diabetes police may conclude that you have forgotten about the effects of junk food on diabetes management. And it will be their job (self-appointed, of course) to remind you, "Y'know, you really shouldn't be eating sweets when you have diabetes!" If you forgot to take your medication this morning, the diabetes police may decide that you must be suicidal and that it will be their responsibility to save you from yourself.

It is a thankless and tireless job, for the diabetes police must be always vigilant, noticing when you are eating (and when you are not eating), when you are checking your blood glucose (and when you are not), and when your blood glucose may be too low (or too high). To keep you in line, they may give you unwanted advice, embarrass you in front of others, or criticize your food choices and other activities. Some people actually enjoy and appreciate such "support," but many feel that such behavior, though well-intentioned, rarely helps. Not everyone has been assigned a member of the diabetes police, but for those who have one, it can be a very difficult experience.

PATRICIA'S STORY

I first met Patricia at a diabetes support group several years ago, the first she had ever attended. She was 45 years old, single, and a successful businesswoman. Patricia had been diagnosed with type 2 diabetes 5 years earlier, but had been ignoring it for most of that time. When asked what she found most difficult about living with diabetes, her response was immediate: "Peanut M&M's. I know I should be eating better, but I just love chocolate of all kinds. Every night, I eat close to a half-pound of Peanut M&M's." As she continued to explain her fondness for different types of chocolate, I couldn't help but notice that the three women sitting next to Patricia were growing more and more agitated. They finally introduced themselves as Patricia's sisters, and—to my surprise—suddenly began screaming at her.

Patricia and her sisters were very close. They saw or spoke with each other almost every day. While Patricia's sisters adored and respected her in most ways, they were infuriated that Patricia had been ignoring her diabetes and were convinced that Patricia could not control her eating without their constant assistance. As they screamed at Patricia that night, I slowly pieced together the story. Despite all of their support of Patricia over the years, nothing had seemed to help. She continued to gorge on chocolate and had slowly been becoming heavier and heavier.

To be honest, Patricia did have a significant problem with binge eating, especially when it came to chocolate. However, the sisters had developed a singularly ineffective approach to helping Patricia with her problem. At least once a week, the sisters would break into Patricia's house and check her cabinets and closets for Peanut M&M's, cookies, and any other chocolate products. When they found any, they threw them away. At church on Sunday, one sister would distract Patricia while the others searched through her purse. When they found any candy bars (which they found *every* Sunday), they would rant and rave at her.

Unfortunately, none of this actually helped. Patricia simply became more adept at hiding her sweets while feeling increasingly ashamed as well as angry at her sisters. To cope with her feelings, she began consuming ever larger quantities of chocolates. In turn, the sisters became even more concerned and exasperated, and they redoubled their efforts to control Patricia's eating.

OFFICIAL POLICE DUTIES

Stories like this are not uncommon. It is far too easy for such patterns of mistrust and anger to develop—between husband and wife, between friends and family members, between parents and children. Even worse, despite all the misery generated, the diabetes police almost never succeed at promoting better diabetes care. In fact, as seen in Patricia's story, they usually make things more difficult. The diabetes police have four major duties: observing, blaming, broadcasting, and advising.

Observing

The diabetes police must stay alert to what you are eating. Indeed, their primary belief is that you cannot be trusted to make responsible food choices. At first, they may only study and evaluate your actions silently. Soon they will begin asking questions, such as, "Should you be eating that?" They will covertly observe your use of medications, exercise, and every other detail of your prescribed self-care, just to make sure that you are toeing the line.

If you have had problems with hypoglycemia, the diabetes police will watch you even more closely. Any gesture or comment you make (especially if you are in a bad mood) may lead to that familiar response, "You seem upset, maybe you should check your blood sugars." The underlying message is that you are a weak, fragile person because of your diabetes and that you desperately need the eternal vigilance of the diabetes police to keep you safe from harm and away from temptation. By constantly observing, they are working to protect you from your own actions.

Blaming

When your blood glucose is too high or too low, regardless of the reason, the diabetes police will hold you responsible. If they can arrange it, you will be manacled and brought to a special, soundproof room each time this occurs. They'll shine a bright light in your face, and the interrogation will begin: "What did you do wrong this time?" There are, of course, an endless number of reasons why blood glucose may rise or fall, and nobody knows them all. To the diabetes police, however, there is only one possible reason: you have done something "bad." If you forget to take your medications, if you overeat, or if you choose not to exercise one day, they will reprimand you for taking imperfect care of yourself. In addition, they will remind you, over and over again, about the terrible long-term complications that may occur because of your behavior. The underlying message is that you are incapable of managing your diabetes without the active direction and criticism of the diabetes police.

Broadcasting

The diabetes police will decide whether or not you are being too secretive about diabetes, regardless of your opinion in the matter. It is their responsibility to inform anyone and everyone about your "handicap." Imagine, for example, that you are enjoying a pleasant meal at a local restaurant with some new friends. As the waitress brings the dessert menus, a member of the diabetes police (your spouse, for example) quickly grabs your menu and announces loudly, "Oh, he isn't allowed to eat any of that, he has diabetes." As mortifying as this may be for you, the diabetes police believe that it is their God-given right to keep everyone you know fully informed.

Advising

The diabetes police take every opportunity to explain how you should take care of your health. Sometimes the information provided is just plain inaccurate, such as, "If you would just stop eating sugar, your diabetes would go away" or "If you'd use more willpower, you could control your eating." However, even when the advice is correct ("If you don't start taking better care of yourself, the odds are good that you'll end up with complications"), it is not necessarily helpful.

WHY JOIN UP?

Given how bizarre and unpleasant all this sounds, why on earth would your family and friends have enlisted in the diabetes police? Is it their intention to drive you batty? Are they enjoying the role of policemen that much? Could it be entertaining to treat you like an idiot, a criminal, or both? It may seem hard to believe, but in almost all cases the diabetes police actually want the best for you. Like Patricia's sisters, even when they are yelling at you, they are actually *trying* to be helpful. They just don't know how else to do it.

Working for the diabetes police is hard and unrewarding, and no one enjoys it. Your friends and family probably understand that their ceaseless observing, blaming, broadcasting, and advising is aggravating you, but they are worried that your diabetes management will only worsen if they shirk their diabetes police duties. They may even want to quit policing, but feel trapped. Your loved ones may fear that *they* will be acting irresponsibly, collaborating with you in the denial of your diabetes, if they are not bugging you enough.

To be honest, their concern (though not their behavior) is sometimes justified. Like Patricia, you may often be bingeing on sweets, refusing to see a doctor, or ignoring some other important aspect of your diabetes management. And, like Patricia's sisters, your friends and family may find this terrifying as well as aggravating. However, the concern of your loved ones is sometimes misplaced. An occasional slice of cake does not indicate that you are suicidal or denying diabetes. Nor does it mean that you have done something "bad." When the diabetes police start blaming, observing, broadcasting, and advising, especially in response to truly innocent actions on your part, it can be quite irritating. And regardless of how much effort or how little effort you are putting into your own self-care, the fundamental problem is that an important personal boundary has been crossed. The diabetes police, your loved ones, have forgotten that it is your life and your body.

DIABETES POLICE AND DIABETES CRIMINALS

Why are the diabetes police so spectacularly unsuccessful? All of us have an instinctual need to be independent, to control our own behaviors, and to make our own decisions, especially in regard to health care. When you are pushed around, treated disrespectfully, or looked upon as an untrustworthy child, there is a strong, sometimes unconscious, tendency to do anything possible to assert your independence. This is true even when it means doing something that will hurt you. One of the more polite ways to stay in control is to become secretive about what you are doing, to hide your actions from the diabetes police.

For instance, Patricia never gave in to her sisters' demands to stop eating chocolate; she simply enjoyed it in private. The less polite approach is to refuse to cooperate, responding to the demands of the diabetes police by doing the exact opposite of what was requested. To illustrate, consider the case of the Hamiltons, Robert and Sarah.

At their first appointment with me, Robert and Sarah, married for 15 years, were barely on speaking terms. Robert, a 36-year-old attorney with type 1 diabetes, had begun having trouble with frequent episodes of low blood glucose several years earlier. Since then, he and Sarah had been through several emergency room visits, one serious automobile accident, and numerous hypoglycemic crises (usually in the middle of the night). While Robert was very concerned, it was clear that Sarah had been even more severely shaken by these experiences. In response, she had joined the diabetes police.

Whenever Robert was at home, Sarah would question him almost hourly about how he felt. She would often urge him to have a little juice or something else to eat, and she would demand that he test his blood glucose much more frequently. Robert understood that his wife's intentions were good, but he was aggravated by her ongoing demands. He soon began responding with a sullen, automatic retort, "I'm fine." And the more she kept insisting that he check his blood glucose, the less he would actually check. "There's no need to check," he would growl, "I'm fine" (which he would say even if he didn't feel fine). Consequently, he began having low blood glucose more frequently. This led to more emergency room visits and even a second automobile accident. Sarah became even more upset and demanding, Robert grew ever more uncooperative, nothing improved, and their relationship began to deteriorate.

It is important to remember that Robert and Sarah loved each other and that they were both acting with the best of intentions (though it was difficult to convince either of them to acknowledge this in the other). Robert was struggling to preserve a sense of control over his own life; Sarah was trying to cope with her own anxiety and help Robert avoid hypoglycemia. This story may sound familiar to you, for it is a common trap for couples coping with diabetes. It is as though you and your loved ones have taken on opposing roles in a movie from which you cannot escape: The harder your spouse works at diabetes police activities, the more you begin to act like a diabetes criminal. Neither police officer nor criminal is enjoying the role, yet both feel powerless to stop.

REAL POLICE AND IMAGINARY POLICE

While you should be wary of the diabetes police, you must also be careful about becoming overly paranoid. Remember that not *all* comments from family members are signs of the diabetes police. When your spouse suggests a new low-fat recipe for dinner tonight, it does not *necessarily* mean that he or she is trying to control your life. When your mother asks you about the missing bag of cookies, it does not *necessarily* mean that she is accusing you of being a bad person or of committing a sinful act. When your boss says that you seem a little pale and wonders if your blood glucose is low, it does not *necessarily* mean that he or she considers you to be an irresponsible person. Indeed, for many people, the diabetes police are largely imaginary. In these cases, although they feel watched and blamed by their family and friends, it is just not so.

As an example, consider the case of Roger, a 33-year-old stockbroker with type 1 diabetes. During our first session, he explained to me that he worked very hard to keep his diabetes hidden from his friends and coworkers. Even when he was with his family, he talked about diabetes as little as possible. And he made sure that they never saw him checking his blood glucose or injecting insulin. It was, as he said, "none of their business." The truth was that Roger was afraid. He was especially afraid that if people noticed how high his blood glucose usually was, they would think less of him and might start nagging him about taking better care of his diabetes. To avoid this, Roger simply stopped monitoring altogether. After several years, this led to consistently high blood glucose levels and the early development of long-term complications. Unfortunately, Roger had read the situation wrong.

After several months of counseling, Roger began to let others know about his diabetes. He also started monitoring more regularly, even in front of his family. To his surprise, he discovered that no one was judging him about his blood glucose or about his diabetes. There were no diabetes police in his life.

As a teenager, however, the diabetes police *had* been a big part of Roger's life. He had constantly been blamed and belittled by his parents about his blood glucose. And there had been many, many arguments. Over the years, he had become convinced that others would treat him similarly if given the chance. As an adult, with his parents now nowhere in sight, Roger failed to notice that the attitudes of the people around him were quite different.

Where the diabetes police had once been real, they were now only imaginary. Unfortunately, for many years these imagined police had powerfully influenced his feelings and actions.

MAKING PEACE WITH THE POLICE

How can you recognize the diabetes police and convince them to turn in their badges? Consider the following six strategies:

1. Start a conversation. In as friendly a manner as possible, talk honestly to your diabetes police about your frustrations. Tell them that you understand and appreciate their concern, but that their policing makes you feel awful and that it isn't helping you to manage your diabetes more effectively. If you are having trouble with your eating, exercise, or some other aspect of your diabetes care, you should acknowledge this to your loved ones. But be assertive about letting them know that you must be in charge of any and all plans for change. Remember that the point is not to blame them (there is already enough blame going around), but to make peace with them.

For example, Matthew was a 68-year-old attorney who had been battling with his wife for years about his weight problems and his diabetes. In desperation, he sat down one day and wrote her a long, heartfelt letter. In the letter, he explained how painful all of her critical, insulting comments about his weight had been. In addition, he spelled out his own frustrations about his weight and diabetes. To his delight, his wife came to him and apologized. She explained that she had meant her comments to be helpful and had never realized how much he was bothered by her words. Thanks to Matthew's action, a warm and genuine conversation between loving partners, rather than police versus criminal, was begun.

2. Advertise your own self-care efforts. Even though you might prefer to keep things private, find public ways to show your diabetes police that you are acting responsibly and thoughtfully about your diabetes self-care. For example, you might let your spouse watch you check your blood glucose, then show him or her how you treat high and low results. Also, you might explain to your loved ones about all of the many diabetes self-care tasks that you do, including those you do well and those you are still working to improve. By speaking out in this manner, you will begin to convince the diabetes police what you already know: that you are a trustworthy, responsible adult.

3. Help the diabetes police to be helpful (in a different way). Because they are people who care about you, it may be almost impossible to stop the diabetes police from being helpful. The trick is to redirect their efforts *away* from actions that are driving you crazy and *toward* actions that may actually be of some value. Thus, it will be valuable to explain to your diabetes police, in a tactful manner, about the concrete types of support that might be of real help to you.

How do you do this? Thank your loved ones for their concern about your health, explain that their actions are not helping you to manage your diabetes better, and let them know that there is a *much more effective* way to help you. For example, rather than yelling at you for overeating again, perhaps your spouse would be willing to stock the cabinets with some less fattening snacks or agree to attend a diabetes education class with you. Following this strategy, Robert explained to Sarah that it was not helpful when she argued with him about hypoglycemia. Instead, he proposed a new deal: if she thought he was hypoglycemic and in need of assistance, she should just bring him a glass of juice, without any comment. In exchange, he promised he would drink it—without any argument.

Making use of your own experiences with diabetes, think of creative ways in which your loved ones could actually be of help. Remember that the diabetes police are eager to be of assistance, at least in most cases. By giving them constructive tasks to do, you are taking an important step toward weaning them from their roles as police officers.

4. Clarify areas of responsibility. Arguments about diabetes care often result from confusion over who should be responsible for which activities. Consider the case of George, a 69-year-old retired engineer with type 2 diabetes, and his wife, Betsy. George and Betsy would argue every evening about whether or not George was eating enough vegetables at dinner. The more Betsy pushed George to eat more vegetables, the angrier and less cooperative George would become. The solution is to work together and to reach an agreement that clarifies the different areas of responsibility—in other words, to decide who will be responsible for what.

When Betsy and George tried this, they were able to agree that Betsy would be wholly responsible for getting tasty vegetables prepared and onto George's dinner plate, and George would be entirely responsible for getting his vegetables from his plate into his mouth. This may sound silly, but it works! When both parties can come to agreement, there is an unmistakable sense of relief. In Betsy's case, she felt freed from her aggravation and guilt that she wasn't pushing George hard enough. In George's case, he felt released from his anger and resentment at Betsy for constantly nagging him. In the end, more vegetables got eaten and the diabetes police went into retirement.

5. Take a good look in the mirror. Consider how your own biases and behavior may be contributing to the problem. First, give careful thought to whether the diabetes police in your life are real or imagined. Are you actually being observed, blamed, or hassled about your diabetes? Perhaps, like Roger, you fear that others are blaming you (or about to be blaming you), even though it is not really so.

If the diabetes police are really at work in your life, think about how your own actions may be contributing to this. For example, Robert's "I'm fine" responses (which he would say even if he wasn't fine) only made Sarah more anxious, leading to more policing. Similarly, Patricia kept bringing candy bars to church every Sunday, even though her sisters would search through her handbag each time. Why would she continue to do so week after week? When her sisters became enraged at her, was this a sign to Patricia that they really cared about her? Perhaps she, like Robert, was merely affirming her independence, reminding her sisters each Sunday that no one was going to control her life. Regardless, there can be no doubt that Patricia's actions were contributing to her sisters' policing behaviors.

So consider whether you may have something in common with Patricia and Robert. Might you be taking such poor care of yourself that your loved ones feel that they must join the diabetes police? Of course, the diabetes police are certainly not blameless, but it is important to remember that *both* sides—police and criminal—con-

> ## SIX STRATEGIES FOR MAKING PEACE WITH THE POLICE
> 1. Start a conversation.
> 2. Advertise your own self-care efforts.
> 3. Help the diabetes police to be helpful (in a different way).
> 4. Clarify areas of responsibility.
> 5. Take a good look in the mirror.
> 6. If nothing else works, get professional assistance.

tribute to the problem. Once this can be acknowledged, change can begin.

6. If nothing else works, get professional assistance. When police and criminal have been locked in battle for years, it can be a difficult habit to break. The diabetes police may fear that if they stop policing, your criminal actions will only intensify. You, the diabetes criminal, may fear that if you give in to the demands of the diabetes police, you may lose your freedom. When no change seems possible, ask your health care provider about referral to a mental health professional who is knowledgeable about diabetes. A little help can make a big difference.

Patricia's sisters, for example, could not stop hassling their sister, and Patricia could not stop bingeing on chocolate. In fact, as they explained their story to me, they could not even stop screaming at each other. At the support group that evening, I felt like I was on a low-budget daytime talk show, just waiting for the violence to begin. Once they quieted down, I convinced them to try the following intervention. Over the next week, Patricia and her sisters would meet together each night. For 30 minutes, they would have a "Peanut M&M party," doing nothing else but enjoying Peanut M&M's. There would be no criticism or comments by anyone. Though they were certain I was crazy, they agreed to this experiment.

By the end of the week, with permission now to eat and enjoy what she previously could only sneak, Patricia soon noticed—to her great surprise—that she no longer liked the taste of chocolate. After years and years of Peanut M&M's, she realized that she had had enough. In addition, with her sisters no longer screaming and trying to control her, she found it much easier to really listen to them. She finally recognized how worried they were about her health and, for the first time, began to understand how important it was to manage her diabetes properly. Patricia's diabetes care soon began to improve dramatically.

This particular type of intervention is certainly not appropriate for everyone, but it may give you a sense of how a little outside assistance can help to resolve the struggle between police and criminal. A variety of different counseling techniques are available, all designed to transform your loved ones from diabetes police back to caring friends.

POLICE NO MORE

By using these six strategies, you can disarm the diabetes police. But before taking any action, always remember that the intentions of your loved ones are good. While they may be driving you crazy, your friends and family are actually trying to be of help to you. Your task will be to educate, letting your loved ones know that you must be treated respectfully, like any other responsible adult, and helping them to understand how they can more effectively support you and your self-care efforts. No police and no criminals, wouldn't that be nice? With tact, kindness, and assertiveness, you can succeed.

CHAPTER 15
Working with Your Health Care Team: The Agony and the Ecstasy

For those of you who despise your doctor (or feel that your doctor despises you), I have disturbing news: If you want to manage your diabetes successfully, it is essential that you have a good working relationship with your doctor and other health care providers. With a close partnership, you can obtain the guidance, support, feedback, and inspiration that is often needed to cope with diabetes day after day. When the relationship with your physician is unsatisfying or troubled, problems with your diabetes care and even your feelings about diabetes can occur.

So what about you? Is your relationship with your diabetes health care team as effective as it could be? When you think about your partnership with your doctor, how satisfied or unsatisfied are you? And what exactly should you expect? What is reasonable? What should your doctor expect of you? How common is it for people to become aggravated, frustrated, or disappointed with their health care providers?

In our research surveys, my colleagues and I have found that approximately one-third of people with diabetes report at least mild aggravations or disappointments with their doctors. These include:

- Feeling that they are not receiving clear enough directions on self-care behaviors
- Believing that their doctor is not spending enough time with them
- Believing that their doctor is not taking their concerns seriously enough
- Feeling that their doctor is unfairly blaming them for "cheating" or not trying hard enough
- Feeling that their doctor doesn't really understand what it is like to live with diabetes

It is, however, an odd and consistent finding across studies that patients rarely consider these aggravations to be serious. Compared with the other stresses of diabetes (such as frustrations with the daily regimen, worries about the future, feelings of burnout and depression, and aggravation with friends and family), frustrations with the health care team are almost always *dead last*. These concerns are rated as less distressing than almost any other aspect of life with diabetes. On average, only about 1 in 20 patients report that aggravations with their physician are a serious problem.

WHY DO SO FEW PEOPLE FEEL BOTHERED?

These findings drove me crazy for many years. How could this possibly be true? The medical visit is a huge source of potential aggravation: physicians are often distracted due to their overwhelming schedules, patients commonly complain of feeling rushed and all but ignored, communication problems occur frequently, and personality conflicts are not a rare event. Why are patients not more distressed by their relationships with their health care team? After further investigation, I finally realize that there are two factors that explain these surprising results: people with diabetes are wise and people with diabetes are not *that* wise.

A Wise Perspective

This pattern of survey responses suggests that most patients (including you, perhaps) are managing to keep a relatively mature perspective on their diabetes care. Although they spend 24 hours a day living with diabetes, they accept that their actual "face time" with the physician is quite limited. An average visit may last 15–30 minutes, but rarely longer. If there are four visits per year, this means a total of approximately 2 hours. Two hours! For the remaining 8,758 hours in the year, the person with diabetes is on his own. So even though visits with the health care team may be discouraging or even upsetting, it usually is not—within the larger scope of day-to-day life with diabetes—perceived as a big deal.

A Not-So-Wise Perspective

It seems that most people have fairly low expectations when it comes to their relationship with their physician. For most patients with diabetes, it is so rare to have a satisfying, get-your-questions-answered interaction with their doctor that they no longer expect it. Thus, no one gets particularly upset when it doesn't happen. Worse yet, because of the recent major upheavals in the American health care system, patients are often required to change physicians on a fairly regular basis. With little consistency in health care providers over time, any opportunity for developing a fruitful relationship is all but lost. These days, a visit to the physician is often seen as similar to an appointment with the auto mechanic. If the doctor seems disinterested, forgets to check your feet, does not take the time to review your blood glucose records, or seems too busy to answer your questions—well, that is just the way it is.

Sometimes this perspective can lead to absurd, and sometimes tragic, extremes. Take the case of Rena, a woman I met at a diabetes support group several years ago. According to Rena, her physician had faithfully checked her blood glucose level at each quarterly appointment over the past 8 years. At each visit, the readings were 200 mg/dl or higher. The doctor described this as "borderline diabetes" and recommended only that they continue to watch this. Rena also told him about the increasing numbness in her feet, but he didn't seem concerned. Although Rena knew enough about diabetes to know that something was terribly wrong (for starters, that there is no such thing as borderline diabetes) and that she needed some form of treatment, she had never raised the subject with her doctor. After all, she explained, "My doctor is a good man, and he once saved my life."

WHAT YOU EXPECT IS WHAT YOU GET

When you have driven nothing but old Buicks throughout your life, it is understandable that you might believe that your car's sluggish acceleration is just the way that all cars work. From the perspective of your neighborhood, where everyone drives an old Buick, it seems a natural limitation to how automobiles are built. However, even though you may not know it, Porsches exist! And— wow—what a ride! This analogy holds true when you consider the possibilities for medical care. Even if you are not terribly distressed about your relationship with your health care team, the odds are good that positive change is possible. A more effective and satisfying alliance with your doctor is possible, and such a partnership can dramatically benefit your diabetes care—perhaps even in ways that you have not yet imagined. Consider the following three examples.

Allie's Story

Several years ago, in the course of an ongoing research project, I had the opportunity to interview Allie, a 38-year-old university professor, about her history with diabetes. She had been diagnosed with type 1 diabetes at age 11 and, unlike most of the people I meet, was relatively at peace with her diabetes. Without a severe emotional struggle to distract her, she had been able to carefully and successfully manage her diabetes since age 24. Before that time, however, she had been "at war" with diabetes. For 10 long years (from age 14 to 24), she had battled her diabetes. Refusing to let it control her life, she kept the illness from most of her friends. She ate what she wanted whenever she wanted, took insulin at random intervals, and avoided checking her blood glucose.

Not surprisingly, Allie's experience with physicians during this period had always been unpleasant. As she depicted it, they had tended to be judgmental and strict. They listed all of the many lifestyle changes with which she must comply while reminding her of all the terrible complications that awaited her if she refused to cooperate. Eventually, she decided to stop seeing doctors altogether. Yet something had happened to Allie at age 24, some event that had helped her begin the process of coming to terms with diabetes. What, I asked her, had happened?

I had expected her answer to be something monumental, a life-changing experience that had commanded her attention. Perhaps she had developed some early complication, such as kidney disease, which had frightened her, or perhaps she had decided to have children. But I was wrong. The event that had begun her transformation was, in fact, a small thing. Allie explained what had occurred:

"After years of pressure from my mother, I finally agreed to see a new endocrinologist. I hadn't seen anyone in several years, and the idea of seeing someone now seemed pointless. To my surprise, the doctor I met was different. He seemed interested in me and actually seemed to care. And that's all it took."

Rather than lecturing her, this physician had listened to her story and then merely asked how he could be of help. He appeared to respect her emotional struggle with diabetes, rather than merely dismissing her as "noncompliant." In a kind and respectful manner, he recommended that she begin with a single change rather than many: checking her blood glucose three times a day over the next few weeks.

"And the most remarkable thing of all," she explained to me, "was that he called me the following week to see how I was doing. He actually called me!"

This simple act of caring was, as it turned out, a key experience for Allie. With the help and support of a concerned physician, her whole attitude toward diabetes began to change. Within 6 months, she had begun to make an emotional peace with the illness and had become involved in an intensive diabetes management program. Her average blood glucose level fell almost 200 mg/dl. And it had remained in the near-normal range year after year for the next 14 years, until I had the pleasure of meeting Allie and hearing her story.

I suspect that there are many people like Allie, people whose attitudes toward their health and their diabetes have been powerfully transformed by a relationship with a caring and knowledgeable health care provider. Unfortunately, it is also likely that the opposite is true: that there are many people for whom a discouraging relationship with their physician was the final straw on the camel's back, leading to diabetes burnout. To be fair, Allie's transformation was not solely due to meeting the right physician. Her willingness to see that doctor, to share her story, and to be open to his comments—all of these personal characteristics contributed to the success of their encounter. What mattered most was the relationship. So the moral of Allie's story is not to abandon your physician and begin immediately searching out the "perfect doctor," but to consider what you can do to improve the relationship with your current health care provider. And this may not be as hard as it seems.

When Patients Are Prepared

In the mid-1980s, a research group led by Dr. Sheldon Greenfield convinced a group of approximately 60 patients with diabetes to participate in an unusual experiment. Immediately before their regular clinic visit with their physician, patients agreed to meet with a research assistant for approximately 20 minutes. For half of the patients (the control group), the research assistant merely reviewed important facts about diabetes, complications, and strategies for self-care. For the remaining half (the experimental group), something much more special occurred. The research assistant became a coach, helping to prepare each patient for his or her upcoming doctor visit. The patient was encouraged to consider what medical decisions he thought needed to be reached at this doctor visit and to formulate the specific questions that he wanted his physician to answer. The "coach" also reviewed a series of negotiation skills and other communication strategies with the patient to make sure that his concerns and questions would be addressed. When the patient returned for his next clinic visit (approximately 3 months later), the same procedure was repeated for a second and last time.

When Dr. Greenfield and his colleagues compared the two groups of patients, the results they uncovered were remarkable. Those in the experimental group felt significantly better and enjoyed a profound improvement in blood glucose control over the course of the study. Blood glucose levels in the control group—as expected—did not change at all. In all of the research that has been done to date, there are very few psychological or behavioral interventions of any kind that have promoted such a powerful and positive effect on long-term blood glucose control. In conversations with their doctors, those in the experimental group were more active, asked more questions, and were twice as effective at getting their questions answered as those in the control group. It seems evident that it was this sense of involvement, personal control, and participation in their own health care that was the major contributor to these impressive blood glucose results.

As Allie's story demonstrated, establishing a good partnership with your physician can have an enormous impact on how well you cope with and manage diabetes. Dr. Greenfield's study suggests how to make this happen. Rather than just hoping that you will discover a doctor as terrific as Allie's, you may be able to create one by actively planning for your doctor visits and being assertive about getting your questions answered.

The Secret of the DCCT

To be a participant in the Diabetes Control and Complications Trial (DCCT) was no easy task, especially for those in the experimental arm of the study. The goal for these people, all with type 1 diabetes, was to reach and maintain near-normal blood glucose levels, day after day, for an average of 8 years. On the whole, they were successful, but the amount of personal effort required was often overwhelming, exhausting, and frustrating. How did they manage to succeed? During the study, which ended in 1992, all medical supplies were provided and all participants had access to the finest medical care and guidance. Every month, and sometimes even more frequently, they would consult with the DCCT nurse educator, who would help identify and resolve their diabetes care problems. But what was the magic ingredient that helped the participants to keep up their efforts over the years?

In a recent survey, a group of former DCCT participants were asked about the type of support that they found most helpful. The clear winner was "nondirective" support. Although medical recommendations and guidance were of clear value, what really helped the participants to maintain their motivation over time was the more global sense that the staff, with whom they had frequent contact, was supporting them and rooting for them. In general, the staff tended to work with the participants in a friendly and respectful fashion, helping them to make their own decisions about how to best manage their diabetes self-care. For the participants, the key to success was knowing that there was someone who would help them figure out what to do, rather than telling them what to do.

BUILDING A BETTER RELATIONSHIP

A coherent theme emerges from these three stories. Although you may not feel particularly frustrated or aggravated with your health care provider, taking action to build a better alliance with your physician and other members of your health care team can enrich your diabetes care and can make it much easier to cope with diabetes. An effective relationship does not mean that you and your doctor must be best friends, but it does mean that:

▎ Your doctor is respectful of your point of view (and you are respectful of his).

▎ Your doctor seems interested in your concerns and opinions (and you are assertive about stating them).

▎ In partnership with your doctor, you are actively involved in all treatment decisions.

▎ Your concerns and questions are addressed.

▎ You receive feedback on all tests that are completed.

In an effective relationship, your physician serves as an able guide to good diabetes care, provides ongoing feedback about your health status, helps you to plan and set self-care goals, and even functions as a friendly cheerleader. Of course, the quality of your relationship does not matter if your health care team is not providing you with the best and most professional care. As a first step, this means checking your feet, eyes, blood pressure, lipid levels, kidney function, and glycated hemoglobin levels on a regular basis. And it means providing the most up-to-date treatment recommendations. This may sound like a lot, but—believe it or not—an effective relationship is possible for almost everyone, even though most appointments are terribly brief.

SIX STRATEGIES FOR BUILDING A BETTER RELATIONSHIP WITH HEALTH CARE PROVIDERS

1. Prepare for your visits.
2. Ask about the results of your medical tests.
3. Use the ABC's of effective communication: assertiveness, brevity, and clarity.
4. Be an active participant in deciding about any changes in your diabetes care (especially your self-care).
5. Take the risk of being open and honest.
6. Be aware of the pressures under which your health care team must operate.

So what can you do to develop a truly effective and satisfying alliance with your health care team? Here are six practical strategies that are likely to help:

1. Prepare for your visits. Unlike Dr. Greenfield's study, your doctor's office does not have a full-time coach to help you prepare for your doctor's visit. However, there is no reason that you cannot do this on your own. Before your next appointment, take a few minutes to write down what you would like to cover at that visit, including:

■ information you want to share or highlight (for example, a blister on your foot or a few days of unusual blood glucose readings)

■ significant problems you are facing (for example, it is becoming harder and harder to find the time to exercise)

■ self-care solutions you are considering (for instance, you are thinking that you might join a walking club)

■ questions you would like answered (for example, perhaps you are worrying about possible side effects from your new medication)

Because the time with your physician is so limited, make sure that you limit yourself to only the most important and relevant issues. And don't just *think* about all the issues that you want to address. It is important that you write them down and take your list to the appointment. There is something very powerful in the act of writing such a list. It can help you to organize your own thoughts and to prioritize the many questions and concerns that you want to have addressed. Also, a list is an enormously helpful memory aid. It is easy to get flustered, forgetful, or intimidated in the midst of your visit; referring to your list can help you to avoid getting distracted and keep you focused on your issues of concern.

2. Ask about the results of your medical tests. To develop and maintain a satisfying partnership, you—being one of the partners—need to know what is going on. Most importantly, make sure to ask your physician about the major medical tests that are so essential to good diabetes care (these include regular evaluations for glycated hemoglobin, microalbumin, lipids, blood pressure, and more). You need to know whether these tests are being done a regular basis and what the outcomes of these tests are.

Take the glycated hemoglobin (HbA1c) test, for example. An indicator of your blood glucose levels over the past 8–10 weeks, this blood test provides the most important information about how well you are managing your diabetes. In good diabetes care, glycated hemoglobin levels should be checked two to four times each year. Unfortunately, many people have never heard of this marker, and many physicians still do not have this test done. And of those people who know about glycated hemoglobin and have the test done, few know what their last test result was and what it means.

This is silly. Imagine going to a weight management specialist and neither you nor the physician ever mentioning anything about your weight. If you are not tracking your weight, if you and your physician have no idea whether your weight is rising or falling, how could you ever know whether your efforts are succeeding or not? When it comes to diabetes management, the glycated hemoglobin test is just as important.

Don't be shy about inquiring about test results and their meanings. If nothing else, remember that you paid for these tests! Staying informed about test result information is one of the best ways to become engaged in your own medical care and to forge a true partnership with your health care team.

3. Use the ABCs of effective communication: assertiveness, brevity, and clarity. When your physician seems distracted, busy, or overly focused on his own agenda for your brief appointment, how can you make sure that your concerns are addressed? Soon after your visit begins, be assertive about telling your doctor that you have some medical issues that you need to review with him and want to know when would be the best time to do this (not *if*, but *when*). The secret to being assertive is to be confident, to speak up for yourself while still being polite. Many people are terribly passive in the presence of a health care provider ("She is a very busy woman; I really shouldn't bother her with any of my questions"). They forget that they have *hired* that physician to provide good medical services.

In combination with assertiveness, it is important that you describe your concerns and questions as concisely and clearly as possible. It is sometimes tempting to relate a long, detailed story to your physician ("So that you understand why my blood sugar was so high that evening, let me tell you about the last 30 years of my marriage"), but that may not be the best use of your limited time together. To put it concisely, be concise!

4. Be an active participant in deciding about any changes in your diabetes care (especially your self-care). At the end of the visit, your doctor may conclude by suggesting one or more treatment-relevant actions, such as a change in medication, referral to another specialist, or a recommendation that you check your blood glucose more frequently. At that point, ask yourself these questions:

∎ Do I understand what he is asking me to do?

∎ Do I understand why he wants me to do this (or how it will be useful)?

∎ Am I truly able and willing to do this?

If you don't understand exactly what is being recommended or why, then be assertive about asking. Your doctor may be using unfamiliar medical terms or not speaking as clearly as he should. Too many people leave their medical appointments feeling confused or unsure about how to proceed. They are too uncomfortable to ask for clarification. If you are not certain, for example, whether you are supposed to be taking two of those new pills three times a day or three of those pills twice a day, this could be a very big problem!

Similarly, if the recommendations are too vague, don't be shy about speaking up. Your physician may suggest that you begin a regular exercise program, but what exactly does she mean by this? A walk around the block once a week? A 10-mile run every day? Given your present condition, what is safe and what is dangerous? And why is this being recommended? Is she concerned about your weight, your heart, problems with insulin resistance, or something else? By clarifying the what and why of this particular recommendation, you will have a much better idea about how to proceed and why you should bother.

Finally, it is essential that you consider your ability or willingness to follow your health care provider's recommendations. The worst thing you can do is to politely agree with all suggestions, even when you know you have no intention of following through with them. If your doctor is advocating that you stop eating cookies each evening but you know, deep in your heart, that you have no interest in doing so, then you need to address this immediately. As an equal partner in your own health care, it is best to respond in a manner that is firm but also friendly and constructive:

"Doctor Smith, giving up my evening cookies is a good idea, but I don't feel prepared to do that right now. Instead, I would like to think with you about some other steps I can take to lower my morning blood sugar levels. Perhaps if I started walking each evening or I increased my NPH insulin dosage at dinner. What do you think?"

Many people find this difficult to do, because they fear disappointing or aggravating their doctor. However, your doctor is not your parent. Instead, think of your physician as your secretary of state, who has been hired to present you with wise and carefully reasoned advice. And you are the president. You and you alone will decide what to do with your secretary of state's advice. In other words, please remember that any decision about changes in your diabetes care should result from a discussion between two, equally responsible adults—you and your physician. When you are actively engaged in making all diabetes care decisions with your health care team, you are certain to feel more in control of your health, more satisfied with your health care providers, and more willing to follow through with all recommended changes.

5. Take the risk of being open and honest. It is not uncommon to see physicians and their patients developing a very peculiar way of relating to each other. Like actors in a bad play, the physician takes on the role of the diabetes police (see chapter 14) while the patient becomes the diabetes criminal. It can be a terribly destructive game, and both parties contribute to it.

The physician begins to behave like an angry and demanding parent, chiding the patient for not taking adequate care of his or her diabetes. Unfortunately, a large number of doctors really tend to think this way, presuming that poor self-care occurs because their patients have no willpower, are not frightened enough, or are not intelligent enough (see chapter 2).

In turn, the patient acts like a withdrawn and sullen teenager, often engaging in the most immature of behaviors. He may, for example, choose not to check his blood glucose, "forget" to bring his blood glucose records to his medical visits, or simply fill his logbook with fabricated "good" blood glucose readings (see chapter 7). When patients and physicians are locked into such unpleasant roles with each other, they cannot function as good diabetes partners. Instead, they are only wary and unhappy adversaries.

It would be nice if your doctor would suddenly decide to quit acting like a member of the Diabetes Police, but do you really want to sit around and sulk until that happens? There is no time to waste, and you can start making some changes right now. To repair such a difficult relationship, you must take the risk of acting differently on your next medical visit. If you are capable of acting like a grown-up outside of your doctor's office, then there is hope that you can do so when you are in the office as well. The secret is to become aggressively honest. Rather than hiding your blood glucose records or doing everything possible to avoid talking about how poorly you have been eating, do the opposite! Make your struggle with diabetes self-care the focus of your conversation with your doctor. Without shame, acknowledge where you are struggling, put forward your own suggestions about how you might handle this problem, and ask for help (see the example above about cookie eating).

6. Be aware of the pressures under which your health care team must operate. Gaining a little perspective on your doctor's situation can help you to build a more effective partnership with him. For most physicians, the amount of time available to see each patient is shrinking, while the mass of paperwork is growing. Many physicians can seem overly curt, gruff, or impolite because they are fearful of having to become involved in a lengthy conversation with their patients. This is not necessarily because it would be unpleasant, but because of the time pressures under which they must work.

Finally, it is important to remember that your doctor may not be as well-trained in communication skills as she should be. Some are, some aren't. After all, those people admitted to medical school are selected because of their demonstrated excellence in such fields as chemistry and biology. Whether they had any personal charm, knowledge of basic etiquette, or expertise in human psychology didn't matter very much. To make the best use of this perspective on your health care providers, take the initiative to practice good communication skills (someone has to start!). Become assertive and engaged in your interaction, and maintain reasonable expectations about your physician's ability to respond to your needs and concerns.

Using these six strategies, you can be confident that the next encounter with your health care team will be more satisfying and productive. Remember that the key is preparation. To take the initiative at your next visit, you should be prepared for what you will say and do differently. To begin this process, take a few moments to complete Worksheet 15.1.

By taking this time to consider—in writing—how you can specifically apply these six strategies, you are now more prepared to approach your health care providers in a new, positive manner. As a memory aid, you might want

WORKSHEET 15.1: A LETTER TO MY HEALTH CARE PROVIDERS

To organize your thoughts for the next meeting with your doctor or other health care provider, please complete this brief letter. Leave any parts blank that you wish. Make use of as many of the six strategies as appropriate.

Dear Doctor,

During our brief visit today, I would like to cover the following issues with you:

A. Information that I need to share with you:

1. _____

2. _____

3. _____

B. Significant diabetes-related problems that I am facing:

1. _____

2. _____

3. _____

C. Self-care solutions that I am considering (to the problems described above):

1. _____

2. _____

3. _____

D. Questions I need answered:

1. _____

2. _____

3. _____

to take this worksheet with you to your next medical appointment.

WHEN ALL ELSE FAILS

Unfortunately, there will be times when these six strategies will not be enough. Doctors are like the rest of us: they come in all different varieties. After trying these strategies, if you are still dissatisfied with the relationship with your physician, the problem may have to do with how your two personality styles mix (or don't mix).

Regardless of the cause, when you cannot connect with your doctor and it is negatively affecting your diabetes management, it may be time to move on. Fire your physician and seek out a new one. Please take note of both parts of the last sentence. Some people become so disillusioned with their doctor that they stop medical care altogether (as Allie did for many years). Have hope that you can establish an effective relationship with a health care provider. It may just take a bit of shopping at first, but it will pay off.

While the vast majority of diabetes care is self-care, there can be no doubt that you need a good working relationship with a health care provider. A skillful doctor will serve as a guide (or, as described earlier, as a secretary of state), as a strong supporter of your efforts, and as a safety net when things go awry. Frustrations and aggravations with doctors are common, but by your own efforts to communicate, you can make a big difference.

Life Stresses/Diabetes Stresses

CHAPTER 16
How Stress Influences Diabetes (and What to Do about It)

The day after Kelly's husband moved out, Kelly began eating cheesecake. She had been careful about eating sweets for many years, but Rod's angry departure seemed to open a floodgate inside of her. Cheesecake and more cheesecake—mornings, afternoons, and evenings. She knew that she was rapidly gaining weight and that her blood glucose was soaring, but everything felt completely out of control. She just couldn't stop.

As the company began to downsize, more and more responsibilities were dumped in Leo's lap. Four of his colleagues had been fired and Leo was now required to complete all of their projects as well as his own. Fearful of losing his job as well, Leo stayed mum. He began working ever longer hours, often as much as 70–80 hours per week. And he was struggling—unsuccessfully—to keep up with the demands. His sleep became increasingly fitful, and he began awakening throughout the night with great anxiety about his job and his future. Remarkably, he was managing his diabetes as well as he ever had, but his blood glucose levels started to rise. To compensate, he tried increasing his insulin doses every few days. But his blood glucose continued to rise. Now, 3 months later, Leo was getting scared. His daily insulin dosage had doubled since the downsizing had begun, and his blood glucose levels remained high.

Can life stress have a negative effect on your diabetes? Of course! Kelly's and Leo's stories are not uncommon. Stress can cause blood glucose to rise and can endanger your health. As a busy human being at the beginning of the twenty-first century, you are guaranteed to suffer through stressful times, at least on occasion. So how worried should you really be about stress? And what should you do? To answer these questions, it is important to learn the real facts about stress and diabetes. The story is not as simple as you might think. For instance, if you have diabetes, will psychological stress necessarily cause blood sugars to rise? Well, the scientific research to date points to a rather confusing answer: yes…and no.

YES, STRESS RAISES BLOOD GLUCOSE LEVELS

Field studies (observing people in their own environments) have demonstrated that stress *can* cause blood glucose to rise. Feelings of distress, especially when they are intense and long-lasting, have been shown to promote a marked elevation in glycated hemoglobin levels. For example, after the tragic 1995 earthquake in Kobe, Japan, researchers found that glycated hemoglobin levels among patients with diabetes rose significantly. These findings were most striking in those patients who had suffered the greatest losses, such as a death or serious injury to a loved one or severe damage to their home. Everyday stresses can influence blood glucose as well. Glycated hemoglobin levels are typically higher in people who are struggling with difficult family situations, troublesome conditions at work, or long-standing emotional problems such as depression.

How could stress affect blood glucose in these circumstances? One method is pretty obvious: When life becomes busy and stressful, diabetes self-care is forced to take a backseat. In other words, stress can raise blood glucose because—as in Kelly's case—it can interfere with diabetes self-management. When you are feeling stressed, you are usually preoccupied with what is bothering you. Because you are focused on other critical responsibilities (say, looking for earthquake survivors) or preoccupying emotions (such as grieving about the loss of an important relationship), your ability to manage your diabetes can be overwhelmed.

NO, STRESS DOES NOT RAISE BLOOD GLUCOSE LEVELS

Laboratory studies (manipulating stress levels in controlled environments) have *not* shown that stress consistently causes blood glucose to rise. Oddly, some studies have shown that stress does affect blood glucose (and/or insulin sensitivity), while others show no effect. This remarkable inconsistency is not due to a lack of effort on the part of scientists. Indeed, my fellow researchers have developed some remarkably clever ways to aggravate their subjects.

In one of the best studies to date, participants with type 1 diabetes were asked to speak to a group of psychologists about their life history and their plans for the future. They were told that the psychologists would be analyzing the content and structure of everything they said. Not surprisingly, this procedure was pretty darned stressful. Heart rate and blood pressure rose significantly, there was a marked elevation in the stress-related hormones (including epinephrine and norepinephrine), and the subjects said they felt quite stressed. But blood glucose levels didn't budge! Although many patients with diabetes, as well as their health care providers, believe that stress can cause an immediate rise in blood glucose—and cases like Leo's continue to occur—there is no good body of scientific evidence to support this belief.

WELL ... DOES IT OR DOESN'T IT?

How can the answer be yes *and* no? This can't be that hard to confirm! Does stress influence blood sugars or doesn't it? From the hodgepodge of scientific data that has been collected over the years, I believe the best answer to be as follows:

- Stress can have a negative effect on diabetes self-management, but only for certain people at certain times.
- Stress can have a direct and immediate effect on blood glucose, but only for certain people at certain times.

Effect on Self-Management

If you are significantly distressed over a long period of time, it is likely that you will begin to have problems managing your diabetes (which can lead to higher blood glucose levels). The most probable impact will be on your ability to exercise regularly or, as in Kelly's case, to follow a healthy meal plan. However, diabetes self-care does not worsen in everyone who goes through stressful events.

Many people continue to manage their diabetes success-fully even during difficult times. This means that the var-ious stress-inducing events (the earthquake, the loss of a relationship, the family argument, or the additional work pressures) are not necessarily damaging to diabetes. Instead, it is how you understand and respond to these stresses that is critical.

In essence, the key factor in determining whether stressful events will affect your diabetes self-care appears to be how you cope with stress in your life, not the amount of stress that is occurring. By responding to stress-ful events in a confident, practical manner, you are less likely to feel too distressed or to have your diabetes self-care compromised. Of course, if this style of coping does not come naturally, you will need to learn how to do it (which we will discuss shortly).

Direct Effect on Blood Glucose

Given the confusing evidence from the laboratory studies, several researchers have recently wondered whether there are important differences between people with diabetes in terms of how they respond to stress. The initial results suggest that there may be three biologically different groups of people. One group appears to be "stress-insensi-tive"; their blood glucose levels are not directly affected by stress. In a second group, blood glucose levels rise under conditions of stress. (Leo would likely be a mem-ber of this group.) Surprisingly, there was a third group of people whose blood glucose levels *drop* when they are stressed. In addition, not all types of stress seem to influence blood glucose. It seems that stress only causes blood glucose problems when you feel trapped in the situation or when it feels out of your personal control. So a scary movie is not likely to influence blood glucose (after all, you have chosen to view that movie and you can leave at any time), but a difficult situation like Leo's just might.

The Bottom Line

So can stress influence blood glucose? Absolutely, but there are enough caveats and conditions to leave anyone feeling a little confused. And not even the scientists truly understand this relationship yet. The bottom line is that stress has the *potential* to interfere with your diabetes self-care, which can elevate blood glucose, and to influence blood glucose directly. And the more distressed you are, the more likely it is that your blood glucose will be affected.

DETERMINING YOUR SENSITIVITY TO STRESS

So what about you? To what degree does stress affect your blood glucose? First, consider whether the stresses that you experience day-to-day might have a significant impact. To investigate this possibility in a careful, structured fashion, please complete one or both of the following exercises.

Exercise 1

Over the next 2 weeks, fill out one row of data on Worksheet 16.1 each day. If at all possible, do not skip any days.

To analyze the completed worksheet, you need to have at least 3 days when your stress level was "2" or lower, 3 days when your stress level was "8" or higher, and 3 days when your stress was in the middle range (between "3" and "7"). If you do not, continue to keep daily records

WORKSHEET 16.1: EXERCISE 1

1. Consider the degree to which you feel stressed. Each evening, circle the number that best describes how distressing that particular day has been. If you feel that you have been free from stress on a particular day, circle "0." If the day has been one of the most stressful you have ever experienced, circle "10."
2. Check your blood glucose at least three times each day. You should check in a consistent manner and at consistent times (before breakfast, before dinner, and at bedtime). Ideally, you should try to keep all other aspects of your self-care as stable as possible over this 2-week experimental period.
3. At the end of each day, record your blood glucose average at the end of each row (add the three blood glucose readings together and divide by three).

		Blood Glucose Readings			
Day	Perceived Stress	Pre-breakfast	Pre-dinner	Bed-time	Average
1	0 1 2 3 4 5 6 7 8 9 10	_____	_____	_____	_____
2	0 1 2 3 4 5 6 7 8 9 10	_____	_____	_____	_____
3	0 1 2 3 4 5 6 7 8 9 10	_____	_____	_____	_____
4	0 1 2 3 4 5 6 7 8 9 10	_____	_____	_____	_____
5	0 1 2 3 4 5 6 7 8 9 10	_____	_____	_____	_____
6	0 1 2 3 4 5 6 7 8 9 10	_____	_____	_____	_____
7	0 1 2 3 4 5 6 7 8 9 10	_____	_____	_____	_____
8	0 1 2 3 4 5 6 7 8 9 10	_____	_____	_____	_____
9	0 1 2 3 4 5 6 7 8 9 10	_____	_____	_____	_____
10	0 1 2 3 4 5 6 7 8 9 10	_____	_____	_____	_____
11	0 1 2 3 4 5 6 7 8 9 10	_____	_____	_____	_____
12	0 1 2 3 4 5 6 7 8 9 10	_____	_____	_____	_____
13	0 1 2 3 4 5 6 7 8 9 10	_____	_____	_____	_____
14	0 1 2 3 4 5 6 7 8 9 10	_____	_____	_____	_____

until this has occurred. If you do, examine your average blood glucose level on those days when your stress was very low ("2" or less). Compute the average of those daily blood glucose readings. Repeat the process for those days when your stress was very high ("8" or higher), and then for those days when your stress was in the middle range. Record these numbers below:

- On my highly stressful days, my average blood glucose was _____.
- On my moderately stressful days, my average blood glucose was _____.
- On my low-stress days, my average blood glucose was

_____.

Do you see any pattern across these three categories? If you see a progression in blood glucose levels from high-stress to low-stress days, then it is likely that life stress does influence your blood glucose. The recommendations that follow will be of particular value for you.

If there is no evident pattern, then congratulations! Because of factors related to your biology or your coping style, you may be resistant to the influence of stress on your blood glucose. Of course, there may be other forces at work here that are masking an underlying link between stress and relationships. For example, if your blood glucose levels are all elevated (perhaps due to an inadequate medication regimen), then there may be little room for stress to play a role at this time. If you still suspect that a relationship exists, then you might take a look at your average *prebreakfast* blood glucose across the three levels of stress, at your average *predinner* blood glucose, and/or at your *bedtime* blood glucose. Stress may be playing a role at only one of these time points.

Exercise 2

Another approach for determining your sensitivity to stress is to manipulate your own stress level and observe how your blood glucose levels respond. To complete Worksheet 16.2, you will need to reserve a 30-minute period on 4 consecutive days. It should be the same time each day, and you should try to keep all other factors as similar as possible from one day to the next: timing of your medication, timing and content of your meals, and timing and intensity of your exercise. If at all possible, do not do this late at night.

Day 1. Check and record your blood glucose level before you begin as well as your best estimate of how stressed you feel *at that moment* (Time 1). If you feel completely at ease and relaxed at that moment, record a "0." If you feel as tense as you can possibly imagine, record a "10."

Next, practice a standard relaxation exercise for 15 minutes. If you do not have a form of relaxation that you regularly practice, you might try this one. Your biggest challenge is likely to be staying awake!

WORKSHEET 16.2: EXERCISE 2

Follow the instructions above and on the next two pages. Rate your stress on a scale from 0 to 10, with 0 being completely at ease and 10 being as tense as you can possibly imagine.

	TIME 1		TIME 2		TIME 3	
	Stress	Glucose	Stress	Glucose	Stress	Glucose
Day 1 (Relaxation)	___	___	___	___	___	___
Day 2 (No relaxation)	___	___	___	___	___	___
Day 3 (Relaxation)	___	___	___	___	___	___
Day 4 (No relaxation)	___	___	___	___	___	___

1. Set a timer for 15 minutes and find a quiet place where you won't be disturbed. Lie down on your back on a comfortable surface. You may want to bend your knees, keeping your feet slightly apart. Make sure to loosen your belt or any other restrictive clothing.

2. Place one hand just below your belly button and the other hand on top of your chest. Close your eyes. Imagine the air coming down, down, down into your abdomen, reaching all the way down into your hips. Each time you breathe in, imagine a balloon in your abdomen that is gently filling with air. Your hand will gently rise with each breath in, and will gently fall with each breath out.

3. Although you may notice the hand on your chest rising and falling, the chest will become more and more still as the body relaxes over the course of this exercise. Soon, the only thing moving will be the gentle motion of your hand on your stomach.

4. There is no need to breathe deeply, or slowly, or quickly. As much as possible, allow your body to breathe by itself. You may notice other thoughts and sensations arising, but try to keep your attention on the sensations of breathing, especially the movement of your hand, as much as possible.

When the relaxation exercise is completed, check and record your blood glucose again as well as your current stress level (Time 2). Sit quietly for 15 minutes, and then check and record your blood glucose and stress level a final time (Time 3).

Day 2. Check and record your blood glucose and current stress level before you begin (Time 1). Spend the next 30 minutes engaged in some typical, though sedentary, activity (say, watching TV or reading a book). Check and record your blood glucose and stress level 15 minutes later (Time 2) and then once again at 30 minutes (Time 3).

Day 3. Repeat the exact process from Day 1 (with relaxation exercise).

Day 4. Repeat the exact process from Day 2 (no relaxation exercise).

Changes in stress. If your blood sugars are sensitive to stress, then they are likely to be sensitive to stress management. To interpret your results, first examine whether your stress level decreased from Time 1 to Times 2 and 3 on the two relaxation days. Although your stress may have decreased on the no-relaxation days also, it should have dropped much more on the relaxation days. If this did not occur, you might want to stop at this point and repeat the experiment with another type of relaxation strategy.

Changes in blood glucose. Second, examine the pattern of changes in your blood glucose levels. If you are sensitive to stress, you might expect to see a markedly different pattern on the relaxation days compared to the no-relaxation days. Most typically, you might see little change on the no-relaxation days and a significant drop in blood glucose level from Time 1 to Times 2 and 3 on the relaxation days. However, be alert for other patterns. For example, perhaps your blood glucose levels tend to rise naturally during this time period on no-relaxation days (maybe you are practicing right after dinner). In that case, if you observe no change or very little change in your blood glucose on relaxation days, this would suggest that relaxation has had a strong effect.

STRESS-MANAGEMENT STRATEGIES

After completing the above exercises, you may have a better sense of the degree to which day-to-day stress affects your blood glucose. Whether stress interferes with your diabetes self-management or directly influences blood sugars via hormonal changes, you should consider strategies for minimizing this effect. Five major strategies for coping with stress are listed below. As an experiment, try one or more of these for several weeks and see for yourself whether your feelings of distress lessen, your ability to manage diabetes improves, or your blood glucose levels become more stable.

1. Begin a regular exercise program. Numerous studies have shown that regular aerobic exercise, such as walking, swimming, or bicycling, reduces the impact of stress on the mind and body. In comparison with couch potatoes, people who exercise regularly are able to handle the stresses of life much more easily. And the amount of time and effort does not have to be daunting. A brisk 15- to 20-minute walk each day, for example, could have a quite positive influence on your stress level. Of course, exercise will benefit your diabetes management as well. So get started! And if you want more suggestions, check chapter 8.

FIVE STRATEGIES FOR OVERCOMING STRESS

1. Begin a regular exercise program.
2. Make a friend.
3. Take a break every day.
4. Challenge your automatic way of thinking about stress.
5. Avoid the dangerous approaches to stress management: drugs and alcohol.

---

2. Make a friend. There is scientific evidence that those people who have good support and love in their lives are also resistant to the damaging influence of stress. In fact, even owning a pet seems to do the trick for many folks. Makes sense, doesn't it? When you feel connected to others, when you feel cared for, when you have some-one to confide in, when you feel part of a loving family or community, it can be easier to keep the stresses of daily life in perspective. Life may then seem less overwhelming. Recent research has even pointed to a direct link with the body: people who feel more connected to others seem to be less biologically reactive to stressful events than lonely, isolated people. For instance, blood pressure does not rise as high and the body's major stress hormones (such as epinephrine and cortisol) do not respond as strongly.

So if you feel more lonely or isolated than you would like to be, think about taking the risk to make a good friend. This could mean repairing a damaged relationship with a loved one or reaching out to deepen the relation-ship with someone you would like to know better. Or it may be time to make some new friends. In any case, make the commitment to take some action that will drive things along in the right direction. Try inviting a neigh-bor over for a cup of coffee, asking one of your workmates to join you for lunch, or joining a new club or organiza-tion. And don't forget that the right kind of friendships can also make it easier to handle the many hassles of liv-ing with diabetes (see chapter 13).

3. Take a break every day. Practicing a structured relaxation exercise every day can protect you against the negative effects of life stress. In addition, there is some evidence that daily relaxation practice might have a direct, positive impact on long-term blood glucose management. There are many different forms of relaxation exercises. These include self-hypnosis, biofeedback, meditation, and progressive muscle relaxation. And any of these techniques is likely to promote beneficial changes, both physical and mental, that reduce stress. Please note that watching TV is *not* a structured relaxation exercise! Relaxation practice is an active, not passive, pastime.

My personal preference is the meditation approach. In fact, the belly breathing exercise introduced in Exercise 2 above is an introductory meditation exercise. Meditation does not mean that you have to wear white robes, change your religion, or fly to the Himalayas. At its core, meditation training is about learning how to focus. Meditation exercises can be practical and portable, and they are remarkably effective in quieting the mind and body. If you are interested in learning more about meditation strategies, please pick up a copy of *Full Catastrophe Living*, by Jon Kabat-Zinn.

4. Challenge your automatic way of thinking about stress. Although life stress is unavoidable, feeling distressed is not. *The critical ingredient is how you interpret and respond to what has occurred.* A difficult event may be perceived as burdensome and depressing to one person, but seem like an exciting, challenging opportunity to another. In fact, one recent study found that glycated hemoglobin levels are elevated during stressful times, but only in those people who tend to respond to stress more emotionally (especially with anger). Thus, if you adopt a more stoic, problem-solving approach to stress, your diabetes management may be less likely to be disrupted during tough times. Of course, changing your habitual style of coping is not easy, since it is typically based on a way of thinking that is deeply ingrained and all but automatic. The best approach to change is to carefully examine and begin challenging your innermost responses to stressful events.

When Kelly, for example, began to investigate her own feelings, she realized how doomed and frightened she felt. She felt certain that she was going to be alone for the rest of her life. Eating cheesecake was her only way to soothe herself and to hold these terrible feelings at bay. Upon deeper reflection, however, she recognized how irrational this was. There was no real reason to believe that her future would necessarily be so lonely. Understandably, she was feeling miserable, but she was far from powerless to influence the next chapters in her life.

In general, you can be successful when you are able to reframe your thinking in such a way you remember that— no matter how stressful your circumstances may be—you are not helpless to effect change. Stressful events may be terribly disruptive, but you can always regain at least a little control over your life (see chapter 18).

5. Avoid the dangerous approaches to stress management. Sadly, many people become dependent on ways of managing stress that don't work; in fact, these approaches tend to aggravate the situation and cause even more stress. Excessive use of alcohol or mind-altering drugs, for example, may be a temporary escape from stress, but it solves nothing. It is also a surefire method for producing more distress in the long term. In addition, because of the many side effects of such abuse (such as interfering with your ability to get deep, restful sleep), the mind and body are likely to become even more sensitive to stress, and more miserable, as further stresses arise. Once you add in the many negative effects of alcohol and drug abuse on diabetes management, you can see that this approach to managing stress is just plain stupid.

Consider the ways you handle stress and how well they actually work. Do you typically become irate and irrational when life becomes stressful? Do you isolate yourself? Do you turn to junk foods for solace? If you rely on these or other types of coping that don't really help you to manage and resolve your life stresses, try something else—such as one of the strategies detailed above. Try anything else!

PUTTING THE STRATEGIES TO WORK

By using strategies such as these and keeping your sense of humor, you are likely to be able to manage the big and little stresses of life. You may also now have a better sense of when and how stress can affect your own diabetes management. One of the important lessons of this chapter is that stress can influence blood glucose, but only in certain people and on certain occasions. It can be tempting to blame every high blood glucose reading on stress (after all, it is a convenient excuse), but this is not always right or helpful. When stress is wreaking havoc on blood glucose, however, making the effort to reduce life stress can pay large dividends.

Kelly reached out to reestablish her friendship with several old chums, began to exercise each day, and as described above, took the time to examine and challenge her automatic thoughts about what had occurred. As a result, she was soon able to give up her daily cheesecake binges and move on to explore her new role as a single woman. Her blood glucose levels began to fall. And to her great pleasure, her weight began to drop as well.

Leo decided to begin a daily relaxation practice. This helped him to feel somewhat less overwhelmed and began to have a positive impact on his blood glucose levels. More importantly, he started to share his feelings with his wife (which he had been avoiding). This helped him to gain an important new perspective on his situation. He realized how unreasonable and impossible his job had become and that it was essential that he confront his boss. To his surprise, his boss responded quickly to lighten Leo's workload. Soon thereafter, Leo's insulin requirements began to fall back dramatically.

Stress can make it more difficult to manage diabetes, but the goods news is that there are ways to handle stress that really work. By trying one or more of the strategies suggested above, you may improve the quality of your life—and your diabetes management. Not a bad deal!

CHAPTER 17
Worrying about Hypoglycemia

Alow blood sugar, a reaction, a hypoglycemic episode— whatever term you use, it is never an enjoyable experience. When your blood glucose gets too low (for most people, this usually means under 60–70 mg/dl), a series of bodily reactions begin to take place that can leave you feeling sweaty, weak, shaky, light-headed, confused, or even worse. At the least, hypoglycemia (low blood glucose) is a nuisance. At worst, it is downright dangerous.

Hypoglycemia is also a common experience. If you are living with type 1 diabetes, hypoglycemia is—unfortunately—a fact of life. For those with type 2 diabetes, especially those on insulin or sulfonylurea medications, hypoglycemia may be familiar as well. Hypoglycemic events are more widespread among those who are taking insulin and occur more frequently in those who are intensively managing their blood glucose. Overall, hypoglycemia is pretty darned common for those with type 1 diabetes and fairly infrequent for those with type 2. However, remember that these are just averages; it varies greatly from person to person. While some people have reactions daily or even more frequently, many have *never* had such an experience.

Depending on the occasion, hypoglycemic episodes can be uncomfortable, aggravating, embarrassing, exhausting, frightening, or even deadly. Remarkably, they seem to occur at the worst possible times: in the middle of an important business meeting, at a crucial moment during a first date, while driving home during a snowstorm, or halfway through your evening jog. Consider the following tales of two diabetes veterans, Jim (type 2) and Alice (type 1).

Jim was almost a mile from home before he realized something was wrong. He had taken his three grandchildren for a long afternoon walk and was pushing the youngest along in the stroller. He suddenly began to feel weak. His heart was pounding, and soon he was sweating profusely. "Oh no, not a reaction, not now," Jim thought, "I didn't bring anything to eat." Jim became increasingly panicked. He worried that he wasn't going to be able to get his three grandchildren, or himself, safely home. With his adrenaline pumping and his symptoms intensifying, he quickly turned and began the long walk home. He was frightened out of his wits, but he worked hard to stay as outwardly calm as possible so as not to scare the children. With great effort, he made it home, where he proceeded to eat almost everything in his refrigerator and finally collapsed into a deep sleep.

Ron was quite surprised when he woke at 3:00 A.M. to find his wife, Alice, pacing at the foot of the bed. Silently and intently, she trod back and forth, back and forth. Ron watched in amazement for several minutes before asking, "Honey, what on earth are you doing?" After a few moments of silence, Alice replied, "Please don't interrupt me; I am looking for my toothbrush." Ron continued to watch her pace for several more minutes before he realized what was occurring. "Honey, I'd be glad to join you in your search for the toothbrush, but I think we should check your blood sugar first."

Though irritated by his request, Alice agreed. A reading of 34 mg/dl confirmed Ron's suspicion, and he hurried downstairs to get a glass of orange juice. By this point, Alice was becoming more confused, and she refused the orange juice. "I can't drink that stuff, I can't," she protested, "I have diabetes." It took some arguing, but Alice finally gave in. After another hour of further monitoring and snacking, Alice was fully recovered and the exhausted couple was finally able to return to bed.

THE THREE TYPES OF HYPOGLYCEMIA

If such events were a daily or even weekly occurrence for Jim or Alice and Ron, they all would probably have gone crazy by now. Luckily, dramatic episodes such as these are rarely that frequent. But how common are hypoglycemic events? There are three different types of reactions to consider:

- severe hypoglycemia
- commonplace hypoglycemia
- stealth hypoglycemia

Severe Hypoglycemia

An episode, such as Alice's, that is so disabling that you need help from others to recover is referred to as "severe hypoglycemia." While this can happen to anyone with diabetes, people with type 1 diabetes are at a much higher risk than people with type 2. The results from the Diabetes Control and Complications Trial (DCCT) suggest that if you have type 1 diabetes and are involved in intensive treatment (aiming for blood glucose levels in the mid-100s or lower), you are likely to suffer a severe episode, on average, once every 18 months. If you are managing your diabetes in a less intensive manner, a severe episode may occur, on average, only once every 5 years. Please be aware that these are conservative figures. The DCCT made a point of avoiding any patients who had a history of problems with hypoglycemia. Therefore, the actual risks may be higher.

In contrast, if you have type 2 diabetes, the risk of severe hypoglycemia is low. Whether you are taking insulin or oral medications, there is only a 1–2% chance of such an occurrence over the next year. In fact, in a recent study of almost 600 patients taking oral medications only, there was just one severe episode during 3 years of observation.

Commonplace Hypoglycemia

A mild or moderate episode, such as Jim's, that you are able to treat on your own is often referred to as "commonplace hypoglycemia." In a typical week, those with type 1 diabetes average about two episodes of mild to moderate hypoglycemia. Thus, they can expect to have *thousands* of such episodes during their lives. Thousands! Episodes are typically much less frequent for those with type 2 diabetes. One study found that just one-third of insulin-using type 2 patients experienced a hypoglycemic episode over a 3-year period. For those taking oral medications only, these occurrences are even more rare.

Stealth Hypoglycemia

Episodes that you never notice can probably be best described as "stealth hypoglycemia." In type 1 diabetes, this is believed to be quite common, especially during sleep. About one-third of patients with type 1 diabetes may suffer such episodes on a regular basis. It is important to uncover these occurrences because they can lead to significant problems. These include reduced hypoglycemia awareness (discussed below), unexplained fatigue, and—in rare instances—damage to the brain. Little is known about stealth hypoglycemia in type 2 diabetes, but it is probably fairly rare.

WORRY CAN BE HARMFUL

Not surprisingly, many people worry about hypoglycemia. Some become so anxious that it severely affects the quality of their lives as well as their ability to manage their diabetes. If you are worried about hypoglycemia, you are not alone. In recent surveys, my colleagues and I found that

- About half of all people with diabetes fret, at least to some degree, about hypoglycemia.
- Among patients with type 1 diabetes, approximately 25% report that worrying about hypoglycemia is a serious problem for them.
- Among patients with type 2 diabetes, approximately 8% report that worrying about hypoglycemia is a serious problem for them.

This chapter is primarily for those people who are anxious about hypoglycemia. But it is also for their loved ones. Family members often worry about hypoglycemia as well. It is not uncommon, for example, to meet spouses who have become so concerned about hypoglycemia, especially during the nighttime hours, that they develop chronic insomnia or other sleeping problems. When hypoglycemia is occurring frequently, this can also set the stage for ongoing family arguments (see the story of Robert and Sarah in chapter 14).

Remarkably, the amount that you worry has little to do with how frequently you have hypoglycemia. If you have had even one episode that was frightening, unpleasant, or embarrassing, you may now be anxious about the possibility of it happening again. In fact, you may be apprehensive about hypoglycemia even if you have never had a blood glucose reading under 150 mg/dl. Anxiety is always about the future, about what could happen.

As worrying intensifies, it can develop into panic or fear. And fear of hypoglycemia can wreak havoc in your life:

■ Many people who are frightened about hypoglycemia decide to keep their blood glucose elevated at all times. They may cut back on their medications, give up exercising, and/or change how they eat. Of course, this is a costly mistake because it increases the risk of long-term complications in the future. The only benefit is that hypoglycemia will be less likely to occur, which does help them to feel less anxious.

■ Eating habits can also deteriorate. To avoid even the possibility of hypoglycemia, some people develop a pattern of eating constantly. Others respond to even the mildest symptoms of hypoglycemia with eating binges. Feeling uncertain about whether or not the reaction will worsen, they eat and eat until the hypoglycemic symptoms subside. I remember many years ago watching a fearful friend who, noticing that he was beginning to shake and sweat ever so slightly, raced to the nearest vending machine and frantically proceeded to empty it of *all* candy bars and then to eat them as quickly as possible.

■ Fearing hypoglycemia, many people become so watchful and worried that they severely restrict their activities. They may be afraid to travel, to drive, to exercise, or even to stray too far from their homes.

WHY WORRY?

Fear of hypoglycemia is about losing confidence in your body, worrying that you might have a serious reaction at any moment. This can happen to people with type 1 *or* type 2 diabetes. Fear of hypoglycemia is about feeling out of control. In your innermost thoughts lurks the belief, "I just can't take this body anywhere! I have no idea what it might do next!" When you lose faith in your body to transport you safely from place to place or to function properly in important situations, it is not surprising that your attitude toward diabetes care changes.

There are four major factors that may contribute to excessive worry about hypoglycemia:

1. Your ability to feel the warning symptoms of hypoglycemia has weakened. The typical warning signs of hypoglycemia include symptoms such as shakiness, sweating, and heart palpitations. These are known as "neurogenic" signs and occur as a consequence of the body's release of epinephrine, one of the major stress-related hormones. Unfortunately, approximately 25% of people with type 1 diabetes no longer experience these warning signs like they once did. For most of these people, there are no obvious warnings that hypoglycemia is approaching at all—no shakiness, sweating, or any other noticeable sign.

This problem is often referred to as "hypoglycemic unawareness," but this name is misleading. Almost no one ever becomes truly unable to notice hypoglycemia; it may just become harder to do than it used to be. A more accurate term is "reduced hypoglycemic awareness."

People with this problem often don't notice that their blood glucose level is dropping until it is already quite low (as low as 30 mg/dl or even lower). At this point, their thinking or even their muscle movements may be seriously impaired; thus, they may be unable to stop what they are doing (say, driving a car) or treat the reaction on their own. As you can imagine, this can be a highly dangerous situation. Of the many people I have met with reduced hypoglycemic awareness, most have encountered difficult problems: car accidents, terrible fights with their spouses, trips to the emergency room, and more. Not surprisingly, most have become vigilant about their blood glucose and quite apprehensive about hypoglycemia.

For many years, it has been widely believed, even among medical professionals, that reduced hypoglycemic awareness is a natural consequence of many years with diabetes. They believe that it just happens, and there is nothing you can do about it. As it turns out, this is not necessarily true. Thanks to recent research, we now know that there is plenty of good news. As we will discuss below, the challenge of reduced hypoglycemic awareness can be met.

2. You have confused the sensations connected to hypoglycemia with the sensations associated with the experience of fear. The signs that warn you of hypoglycemia are very similar to what happens in your body when something frightens you. A racing heart, for example, could occur when someone surprises you from behind *or* when your blood glucose starts to drop too low. These signals can become mixed or confused: you can't be sure whether what you are feeling is fear, hypoglycemia, or both. When this occurs, even a mild reaction can trigger a major fear response. Although the hypoglycemic episode may be a little scary ("Uh oh, my blood sugar is low and it may be dropping"), the misinterpretation of these bodily cues as fear intensifies this response dramatically ("Oh my God, I'm having a reaction. I'm in very big trouble. I better eat everything in the refrigerator!").

Also, any feelings of fear or nervousness that may occur throughout the day, regardless of what your actual blood glucose level is, may convince you that hypoglycemia is approaching. This is likely to make you feel more frightened, which makes you even more certain that you are hypoglycemic, which makes you feel even more terrified. And the downward spiral goes on. As this pattern continues over time, you may become increasingly oversensitive. Even the most harmless of body sensations (for example, your heart beating faster for a few moments) leads to the same familiar spiral of thoughts and feelings: "This could be hypoglycemia, which makes me nervous. Now that I'm nervous, I notice that my heart is beating even faster, which makes me even more certain that this is hypoglycemia, which makes me even more nervous!"

Worse yet, much of this may be occurring outside of your awareness, so all you notice is that you seem to be having reactions over and over again throughout the day, even though your blood sugars are never actually low. People with this type of problem may end up with chronically high blood glucose (because they are constantly eating in response to reactions that are not reactions) or very sore fingers (because they are checking their blood glucose 20 times a day or even more). Sometimes this worsens into a full-fledged panic disorder, leading to chronic anxiety, and in some cases, to frequent and frustrating trips to the emergency room.

3. You are having difficulty estimating or predicting your blood glucose level, especially when it is low. Even when your neurogenic warning signs are working well, you may still be having problems recognizing hypoglycemia. Indeed, recent research has shown that when people are actually below 70 mg/dl and they are asked to estimate their blood sugar level, they guess that it is much higher (out of the hypoglycemic range) about half the time. Half the time! Because many episodes of low blood glucose are never noticed, this suggests that they are not treated until glucose dips quite low. This increases the chances that more serious problems will arise.

One of the more common reasons for not recognizing hypoglycemia is that you are relying too heavily on the *wrong* cues to warn you that you are low. For example, many people believe that feelings of hunger or fatigue are good warning signs of hypoglycemia. In most cases, they are not. So, one day, you may notice a number of warning signs (shakiness and tingling, for example), but because you don't feel hungry or tired, you dismiss these other feelings. "I can't be low," you might say to yourself, "because I don't feel hungry."

In addition, we now know that the body cues linked to hypoglycemia differ from person to person, sometimes quite a bit. Although you may have been taught to watch out for the "classic" symptoms, your very best warning sign may be quite unique: a trembling of the upper lip, a funny taste in your mouth, or a peculiar feeling in your legs. Thus, you may fail to recognize hypoglycemia because you are waiting patiently to notice the symptoms you've been schooled to expect (which may never occur) while never noticing the more useful warning signs that are unique to your own body.

There can also be a problem if you rely too heavily, or too lightly, on the cues provided by your diabetes regimen. For example, I remember a young lady who sat in my office and suddenly began sweating and trembling. When I suggested that she might be hypoglycemic, she responded, "I just checked my blood sugar 30 minutes ago and it was fine, so I can't be low." Want to bet?

4. You have experienced a serious and frightening hypoglycemic event. Perhaps you have been taken to an emergency room, suffered a terribly embarrassing moment in public, or been involved in a traffic accident. To feel out of control in this manner can be quite unnerving. And once such an event has occurred, you may be traumatized. You may worry constantly that such an event will occur again. Of course, whereas excessive worrying about hypoglycemia is problematic, worrying in smaller doses is not necessarily a bad thing. It makes sense that you would become concerned after a difficult episode. In response, you would become more careful. Perhaps you would consult with your doctor and work on adjusting your diabetes care so that this would not happen again. Or you would vow always to check your blood glucose level before you get into a car to drive somewhere.

Unfortunately, I have also met a number of individuals who have no sense of apprehension about hypoglycemia at all, despite a history of many severe reactions and frequent trips to the emergency room. Sandy, for example, had been taken to the emergency room so many times that she was on a first-name basis with all of the county paramedics. Still, she didn't feel that hypoglycemia was dangerous; after all, the paramedics had always arrived in time (at least so far). She rarely checked her blood glucose and saw no reason to do so. I only wished she would begin to worry!

Each of these factors can contribute to a loss of confidence in your body, so that you become more and more anxious about hypoglycemia. Such worries can influence your diabetes self-management, even if they are not conscious. In my practice, for example, I remember working with a young woman who snacked on junk food (primarily donuts, chips, and candy bars) throughout the day. Despite her best efforts, she was unable to stop herself for more than a day or two at a time. Consequently, her blood glucose levels were chronically elevated. She believed that she had a serious eating disorder, but after careful evaluation, we realized that the major driving force behind her need to eat was a fear of hypoglycemia. Many times each day she would become suddenly afraid that her blood glucose might be dropping (set off, perhaps, by a minor twitch or some other mundane event). The solution, of course, was to eat, and eat and eat. Despite the power of this fear, it had become such an everyday part of her life that her response was now automatic. She had stopped noticing that the feeling of fear was present.

My colleagues and I recently completed a study where we found that fear of hypoglycemia is particularly high among women with diabetes who regularly omit their daily insulin (a very destructive thing to be doing). A serious eating problem is the major reason why someone begins to cut back on their insulin (see the box "Eating Disorders and Diabetes" on pages 65 and 66 and chapter 6), but worrying about hypoglycemia provides one more excuse to cut back. Fear of hypoglycemia adds fuel to the fire.

HOW MUCH DO YOU WORRY?

Have you ever wondered whether you might be worrying about hypoglycemia more than is reasonable? Or wondered what to do because you are worrying too much about hypoglycemia? In either case, the first step is to determine how apprehensive you really are. To do so, please complete Worksheet 17.1 now.

If your total score on Worksheet 17.1 is 25 or higher, then you are significantly more nervous about reactions than most people. Your fear of hypoglycemia is probably affecting the quality of your life as well as your ability to manage your diabetes. If your score is less than 25, then your concerns probably fall within the range of what is considered to be normal.

OVERCOMING WORRY

If you are significantly frightened about hypoglycemia (a total score of 25 or higher), or even worrying more than seems reasonable to you, take hope. Like many others, you too can regain your personal sense of confidence and comfort. Much of the credit for this good news goes to a hard-working group of clinical researchers at the University of Virginia, led by Drs. Daniel Cox and Linda Gonder-Frederick. After many years of careful study, they have developed a remarkable and successful program called

Blood Glucose Awareness Training, or BGAT. Among other achievements, this program has been shown to help people detect low blood glucose more regularly and to reduce the number of severe hypoglycemic episodes—all without leading to elevated blood glucose levels. As we now consider 12 major strategies that can help you overcome your worries about hypoglycemia, please note that most of what you will read has been adapted from the work of Dr. Cox, Dr. Gonder-Frederick, and their colleagues.

1. Consult with your health care provider. No matter how frustrated you are, a good talk with a physician who is well trained in diabetes may be the most useful step you can take. For instance, if you no longer feel the typical warning signs of hypoglycemia, there are new medical strategies that may help you recover these important cues. Over the past few years, researchers have discovered that a period of just a few weeks without having any low blood glucose levels can restore some of the symptoms for most people. Remarkably, this can be achieved without raising your glycated hemoglobin levels. Thus, through careful planning with your doctor, you may be able to regain your ability to sense approaching hypoglycemia before your blood glucose drops too low.

Even if you are fully able to sense the early signs of hypoglycemia, you may still be troubled by frequent low blood glucose levels. If hypoglycemia seems to be a constant companion, and especially if you are experiencing severe episodes, a thoughtful change in your medication (type, dosage, or timing) or some other aspect of your diabetes regimen may be indicated. This is another good reason why a visit to your health care provider could prove to be valuable.

WORKSHEET 17.1: HOW WORRIED ABOUT HYPOGLYCEMIA ARE YOU?

This questionnaire was developed by Dr. Daniel Cox and his colleagues at the University of Virginia School of Medicine.
Directions: Below is a list of concerns people with diabetes sometimes have about low blood sugar. Circle the number to the right that best describes how often in *the last 6 months* you WORRIED about each item because of low blood sugar.

Because my blood sugar could go low, I worried about:

	Never	Rarely	Some-times	Often	Always
1. Not recognizing/ realizing I was having low blood sugar.	0	1	2	3	4
2. Not having food, fruit, or juice available.	0	1	2	3	4
3. Passing out in public.	0	1	2	3	4
4. Embarrassing myself or my friends in a social situation.	0	1	2	3	4
5. Having a hypoglycemic episode while alone.	0	1	2	3	4
6. Appearing stupid or drunk.	0	1	2	3	4
7. Losing control.	0	1	2	3	4
8. No one being around to help me during a hypoglycemic episode.	0	1	2	3	4
9. Having a hypoglycemic episode while driving.	0	1	2	3	4
10. Making a mistake or having an accident.	0	1	2	3	4
11. Getting a bad evaluation or being criticized at work.	0	1	2	3	4
12. Having difficulty thinking clearly when responsible for others.	0	1	2	3	4
13. Feeling light-headed or dizzy.	0	1	2	3	4

WORKSHEET 17.1: HOW WORRIED ABOUT HYPOGLYCEMIA ARE YOU? *(Continued)*

14. Accidentally injuring myself or others.	0	1	2	3	4
15. Permanent injury to my health or body.	0	1	2	3	4
16. Low blood sugar interfering with important things I was doing.	0	1	2	3	4

Now add up your responses to determine your
TOTAL SCORE: _____

2. **Learn the facts about the warning signs of hypo-glycemia.** The neurogenic symptoms that accompany hypoglycemia occur for an important purpose: they are the body's smoke alarm, alerting us to a danger that must be addressed. However, the true and complete story about hypoglycemia is more complicated.

The neurogenic cues are only one of a number of smoke alarms that each person possesses. As blood glucose drops, other body systems come into play, leading to changes in how you think, move, and feel. The most important of these are known as "neuroglycopenic" signs. These occur when not enough glucose is getting to the brain. Often referred to as "brain sputtering" cues, these symptoms can be very dramatic (suddenly being unable to speak) or quite subtle (having a little trouble concentrating while you are reading).

It was once commonly believed that the classic neuro-genic symptoms occurred long before any signs of brain sput-tering. The thinking was that neurogenic symptoms typically occurred at a blood glucose level of around 70 mg/dl (although this varied considerably from person to person), while neuroglycopenic cues didn't occur until 40 mg/dl or so. Thus, it seemed that neuroglycopenic cues didn't occur until it was all but too late. A typical story would be that of the gentleman who, feeling "a little funny," decided to check his blood glucose and discovered that he was at 25 mg/dl. He sat there, just staring at his meter, while thinking, "Hmmm. I know that this number means something, that there is something I should do. But I have no idea what that could be." Truly, if brain sputtering cues don't occur until blood glucose is this low, then they hardly classify as a good smoke alarm. The house has already almost burned down!

However, this is not the whole story. As it turns out, neuroglycopenic and neurogenic signs actually seem to occur at close to the same blood glucose level. Even at 65–70 mg/dl, your brain is starting to sputter, at least slightly, even if you do not recognize it. In fact, neuroglycopenic cues are the first symptoms to be noticed by some people. And here is the good news: If your neurogenic warning signs become weakened or lost, you still have your brain sputtering signs. Reduced hypoglycemic awareness means that one of your smoke alarms has been damaged, but you have other alarm systems that can be put to good use (see strategy 11).

When it comes to warning signs, there can be large differences from person to person. What is the first thing you notice as your blood glucose drops into the hypoglycemic range? What is your most reliable body cue? As discussed earlier, for some people, it may be one of the neurogenic cues (such as sweating or a tingling sensation). For others, it may be a neuroglycopenic cue (such as difficulty with making change), a change in mood, or even something more unusual. Your best warning signs are likely to be unique to you. However, even when your warning signs are functioning well, you sometimes may not notice them. For example, this can occur if you are feeling very anxious or preoccupied with a task.

3. Respond to a hypoglycemic number, not just a hypoglycemic feeling. Some people believe that you don't need to treat a reaction until you begin to feel symptoms. This is a terrible mistake. On some occasions, a hypoglycemic episode can occur without your noticing the warning signs. So you should be prepared to respond to a low blood glucose reading even when you don't have symptoms. Talk with your health care provider about the actual number at which you should take action. For some people, this might be as low as 60 mg/dl. For others, it might be as high as 120 mg/dl or even higher. Through prompt action, you can avoid bigger problems.

4. Don't delay treatment for hypoglycemia. If you want to avoid severe hypoglycemia, this may be one of the most important things to keep in mind. Many people try to tough out the symptoms of hypoglycemia. They recognize when their blood glucose is low, but they don't treat it until they have finished what they are doing—be it sitting in a business meeting, mowing the lawn, or driving home from work. In the meantime, their blood glucose continues to drop.

Ignoring the symptoms of hypoglycemia is often a way of trying to fight for control: "I'm not going to let diabetes interrupt my daily life or push me around in any way!" But this is a poor battle to choose. The result can be severe hypoglycemia—which can really interrupt your day!

5. Treat hypoglycemia with something that works. To have confidence in your body, you need to know that you can raise your blood glucose level quickly when hypoglycemia strikes. Indeed, there are few things more unnerving than sitting alone, sweating and shaking from hypoglycemia, then consuming a good-sized snack *and still be sweating and shaking!* Most people know that simple sugars, such as honey, milk, orange juice, cake icing, and glucose tablets, are the best foods for raising your blood glucose rapidly. Unfortunately, a common error is the belief that any food with lots of sugar in it will work just as well. Thus, many people use products such as chocolate candy bars to treat reactions. The bad news is that these do not usually work very well.

Chocolate bars contain plenty of simple sugars, but they also have a lot of fat. The large amount of fat slows the body's absorption of the sugars, so there is only a very slow rise in blood glucose. As tasty as a candy bar may be, it is not effective as an emergency food and can end up making you feel even more frightened in the face of hypoglycemia. So choose foods that make you feel better quickly.

6. Always carry a fast-acting carbohydrate with you. Many serious episodes of hypoglycemia happen because people break this simple rule. If you aren't prepared to respond to hypoglycemia, it doesn't matter how much you know. Make sure that you keep hard candies, glucose tablets, or other fast-acting products at work, at home, in the car, and anyplace else you spend time. It is especially important that you carry something with you when you are doing any kind of physical activity (remember Jim's story?). Think of these products as you would your house keys, wallet, or purse: Don't leave home without them!

7. Take action to overcome the "I'm fine" syndrome. The more you feel pestered by friends or family members about the possibility of low blood glucose, the more likely it is that you will ignore their warnings and push them away. Because you, like most people, are probably too polite to scream "Butt out of my business!" you may respond with "I'm fine." The messages, however, are the same: "I will control my own fate, not you."

Unfortunately, you can become so resistant to the comments of others, no matter how helpful they are trying to be ("Honey, your eyes seem a little glazed; maybe you should check your blood sugar?"), that you may automatically reply, "I'm fine," even if you don't feel fine. To assert your own independence in the face of your loved ones' worrying, you may even refuse to notice the warning signs of hypoglycemia. This may lead to more frequent and severe hypoglycemic episodes, which make family and friends even more anxious to be of help, which leads to even more cries of "I'm fine" and possibly more hypoglycemia, and on and on. Sadly, everyone involved in this whole terrible mess has only the best of intentions.

How do you break out of the "I'm fine" syndrome? The most important step is to start an open-ended conversation with your loved ones about your mutual frustrations. For more specific strategies, see chapter 14.

8. Take a breath, especially if you tend to think you are having reactions even when you are not. For most people, a brief relaxation exercise can dampen down physical sensations related to anxiety or fear, but it will have little effect on true hypoglycemic symptoms. As a first step, practice a simple exercise such as the one that follows:

While sitting comfortably in a chair, close your eyes and take a slow, deep breath. When you have expanded your lungs fully, hold the breath in for a few seconds.

Then breathe out as fully as possible and hold the breath out for several more seconds. Once again, a second deep breath, then holding the breath in for a few seconds. Breathe out fully and hold the breath out for a few seconds. Repeat this cycle for a third and final breath. Then open your eyes and notice whether you sense any subtle differences in how you feel, either physically or mentally.

After practicing this exercise on several occasions, you should notice a distinctive sense of relaxation. As a second step, practice this exercise when you begin to have confusing hypoglycemic symptoms. If the symptoms significantly weaken or disappear, it is likely that you were experiencing a false alarm. If the symptoms remain, your feelings may be a true warning sign of hypoglycemia. However, please do not take my word for any of this! This is merely an experiment to try. Check your blood glucose and see for yourself whether this is correct. If so, then continue to practice this simple relaxation episode each time you have puzzling hypoglycemic symptoms. With continued practice over several months, you should expect that the false alarms will happen less and less frequently.

9. Immediately before checking your blood glucose, guess what the number will be. What do you think your blood glucose level is right now? To a large extent, having faith in your body means having at least a rough idea of where your blood glucose level is at any moment in time, especially if it is in the hypoglycemic range. Although it is wise to use your blood glucose meter frequently, you can never depend on it completely. Your fingers could never stand it! There are just too many times during the day when you must make automatic decisions, both little ones and big ones, based on what you think your blood glucose is. For example, "It is probably safe for me to take a nap now. After all, I just ate."

As mentioned earlier, however, research suggests that as many as 50% of hypoglycemic episodes are not detected as quickly as they could be. This is pretty bad. Therefore, an important first step toward regaining confidence is to start guessing—to find out how accurate or inaccurate you really are. Over the next few weeks, try this experiment: Each time you are preparing to check your blood glucose, take a good guess at what your level is. Record that guess in your logbook, right next to your actual reading. Be precise about your guess; don't just estimate that it is "above 100," "about 80," or something similar. Also, make sure that you record your guess before you lance your finger. This is important because some people are—amazingly— fairly good at estimating their blood glucose level based on the color of their blood. Once you have guessed and recorded at least 50–60 blood glucose levels, you will be ready to discover what kind of a guesser you are.

10. Determine how well you recognize your hypoglycemia (and learn about the specific types of mistakes you make). Once you have recorded at least 50–60 blood glucose guesses, please complete Worksheet 17.2.

Your scores on Worksheet 17.2 will place you in (or close to) one of four groups:

▌ **Good guessers.** If your percentage of correct hypoglycemic guesses is high (50% or higher) and your percentage of incorrect guesses is low (20% or lower), then you are pretty good at detecting hypoglycemia. For some people, discovering that they fall into this category is tremendously reassuring. They realize that they can have much more confi-

WORKSHEET 17.2: HOW WELL DO YOU RECOGNIZE HYPOGLYCEMIA?

How many of your actual low blood sugars were you able to identify CORRECTLY?

▮ Of the 50–60 blood sugars that you guessed, how many of the ACTUAL blood sugars were lower than your hypoglycemic number (from strategy 3, the number below which you would take action)? In other words, how many low blood sugars did you actually have?   Score 1_____

▮ Of those that were ACTUALLY less than your hypoglycemic number, how many did you GUESS were under that number?   Score 2_____

▮ Compute your PERCENTAGE OF CORRECT HYPOGLYCEMIC GUESSES:
a. Score 2 x 100 = Score 3_____
b. Score 3 ÷ Score 1 = Percentage of Correct Guesses

_____

How often did you INCORRECTLY guess that a low blood sugar was occurring?

▮ Of the 50–60 blood sugars that you guessed, how many of the ACTUAL blood sugars were higher than your hypoglycemic number?   Score 4_____

▮ Of those that were ACTUALLY higher than your hypoglycemic number, how many did you GUESS were under that number? Score 5_____

▮ Compute your PERCENTAGE OF INCORRECT HYPOGLYCEMIC GUESSES:
a. Score 5 x 100 = Score 6_____
b. Score 6 ÷ Score 4 = Percentage of Incorrect Guesses

_____

dence in themselves and in their body than they thought possible. Still, serious mistakes could always happen (or may have already happened), so it is important to consider how you can make your guessing ability even more effective.

- **Nondiscriminating guessers.** If your percentage of correct hypoglycemic guesses is high (50% or higher) but your percentage of incorrect guesses is also high (50% or higher), then you tend to guess that you are low, regardless of what your blood glucose level really is. How nerve-wracking! You may be confusing the symptoms of fear with the symptoms of hypoglycemia. Thus, you may be panicking about reactions even when you are not low. Your goal should be to become a more accurate and *discriminating* guesser.

- **Poor guessers.** If your percentage of correct hypoglycemic guesses is not high (lower than 50%) and your percentage of incorrect guesses is also not high (20% or lower), then you are not very good at detecting hypoglycemia. Luckily, you are not tending to guess you are low when you are not, so you are probably not excessively watchful for hypoglycemia. Still, your job will be to become more accurate at guessing.

- **Mixed-up guessers.** If your percentage of correct hypoglycemic guesses is not high (lower than 50%) and your percentage of incorrect guesses is high (50% or higher), then you are probably driving yourself crazy! You often think you are low when you are not, and you often think you are not low when you really are. Of the four groups, you have the toughest job of all: learning to more accurately estimate when hypoglycemia is present *and* when it is not present.

Consider the case of Robert, whom you met in chapter 14. After many months of frequent hypoglycemic episodes, Robert came to an agreement with his physician that any number under 90 mg/dl would be considered low and he would take action. After completing the guessing experiment and Worksheet 17.2, Robert was sobered to learn that he fell into the "poor guesser" group. He was only recognizing one-third of his low blood glucose levels. To his dismay, it was now clear that his wife's fears were well-grounded. On the positive side, he was only rarely making the mistake of thinking he was hypoglycemic when he was not. To regain his confidence, it was essential that Robert's initial goal be to redevelop his ability to detect hypoglycemia before it became serious. How could he, or you, regain this skill? Well, read on.

11. Discover your body's unique smoke alarms. One of the techniques that can help you to become more effective at

---

TWELVE STRATEGIES FOR OVERCOMING YOUR WORRIES ABOUT HYPOGLYCEMIA

1. Consult with your health care provider.
2. Learn the facts about the warning signs of hypoglycemia.
3. Respond to a hypoglycemic number, not just a hypoglycemic feeling.
4. Don't delay treatment for hypoglycemia.
5. Treat hypoglycemia with something that works.
6. Always carry a fast-acting carbohydrate with you.
7. Take action to overcome the "I'm fine" syndrome.
8. Take a breath, especially if you tend to think you are having reactions even when you are not.
9. Immediately before checking your blood glucose, guess what the number will be.
10. Determine how well you recognize your hypoglycemia (and learn about the specific types of mistakes you make).
11. Discover your body's unique smoke alarms.
12. Learn more about Blood Glucose Awareness Training (BGAT).

recognizing hypoglycemia is to begin identifying those subtle signs (which, in many cases, are unique to you) that accompany low blood glucose. These may include neurogenic symptoms, changes in mood, and/or signs of brain sputtering. The best approach is to keep a careful and detailed diary of your blood glucose readings for at least several weeks. Building on strategy 10, record your blood glucose guesses (along with your actual meter readings), and in addition, indicate any bodily or mental sensations you may be noticing at the time. After several weeks, you can then investigate the information that you have collected in any of a number of different ways.

For example, give special attention to those times when you guessed correctly that you were hypoglycemic. Were there any bodily or mental sensations that helped you to guess right? For many people who are struggling with reduced hypoglycemic awareness, focusing on the subtle signs of brain sputtering may be especially valuable in the detection of even mild hypoglycemia. For instance, some people begin to recognize subtle changes in their *motor* skills as their blood glucose drops into the hypoglycemic range. Consider the following examples:

▪ After many weeks of careful record keeping and observation, a carpenter noticed that he was fumbling with nails when his blood glucose dipped below 65 mg/dl.

▪ An administrative assistant realized that she was hitting the computer keys slightly harder.

Others become aware of changes in their *mental* abilities:

▪ A housewife noticed that she had trouble concentrating while reading when her blood glucose dipped below 60 mg/dl.

■ A salesman realized that he was occasionally having difficulty finding the right word when talking.

As brain sputtering begins, many people adapt quickly and automatically. So it can take considerable effort to notice the signs. The administrative assistant, for example, never realized that it was becoming increasingly difficult to type accurately. Instead, she began to notice her automatic response: she was hitting the keys harder and harder. It is much easier to notice the early symptoms of your own brain sputtering when you are performing a challenging task, either a physical task (like sewing), a mental task (like reading), or a combination of the two (like flying the space shuttle). When you are watching television or doing a routine task, it is much more difficult. Thus, if you cannot detect any signs of brain sputtering when your blood glucose dips into the hypoglycemic range, look for ways to challenge your brain. A teacher, for example, decided to do his times tables for the number 12 (12, 24, 36, 48, 60, and on) immediately before he checked his blood glucose for several weeks. He discovered that he was significantly slower at this task when he was even mildly hypoglycemic. With this realization, he began to recognize similar warning signs that helped him to notice hypoglycemia before it became too serious.

As you discover one or more smoke alarms that are reliably linked to your low blood glucose—be they changes in mood, subtle neurogenic signs, brain sputterings, or something else—you can begin to use them to become an increasingly accurate guesser of early hypoglycemia. Of course, this will not and should not take the place of blood glucose monitoring. Rather, it can help you to identify additional moments when it may be important to check your blood glucose level.

12. Learn more about Blood Glucose Awareness Training (BGAT). Although you can improve your ability to detect hypoglycemia, it is not necessarily easy. Even the detection of useful smoke alarms can be difficult and time-consuming. BGAT is a comprehensive, multi-session program that guides you in the systematic development, evaluation, and application of the information you can derive from your blood glucose diaries (which includes your actual blood glucose readings, your corresponding guesses, accompanying mental and physical sensations, and more). This involves observing and learning about all of your body's potential smoke alarms as well as harnessing the knowledge of your diabetes regimen to estimate and predict what your blood glucose is most likely to do—for example, discovering how your early evening exercise may be affecting your blood glucose throughout the night. Because half of all severe hypoglycemic episodes occur during sleep, being able to accurately predict how your blood glucose will change in the near future is as important as being able to accurately guess what your blood glucose level is right now.

To detail the entire BGAT program is beyond the scope of this book, but if you are interested in learning more about the program, ask your physician or local diabetes educator. You may also contact Drs. Cox and Gonder-Frederick directly at the University of Virginia Medical Center, 804-924-5316.

CHAPTER 18

When Good Actions Don't Lead to Good Results: The Blood Sugar Fairy and Other Uplifting Tales

Once upon a time, diabetes was the easiest disease in the whole world to manage. With minimal effort, every child or grown-up with diabetes was able to achieve perfect blood glucose levels all the time. Everyone ate well, exercised regularly, and enjoyed themselves while they did so. Almost no one ever experienced a blood glucose level that was too high or too low. Blood glucose monitoring brought nothing but good news. So no one ever got upset or disappointed, and families never argued. On rare occasions, blood glucose levels would drop steeply or skyrocket, but there was never any confusion about why this had occurred. An extra piece of pie last night, an unusual medication, too little exercise this morning—it was always easy to find the problem and to resolve it quickly. Diabetes made sense. Diabetes could be controlled. It was a wonderful, easy, and happy life for all ... until the coming of the Blood Sugar Fairy.

It took many years to discover that it was the Blood Sugar Fairy, a tiny and invisible pixie, who was the cause of the consternation and chaos that followed. No one ever discovered where she came from, though some guessed that she was a distant relative of the Tooth Fairy (from the cranky, dysfunctional side of the family, of course). It was the Blood Sugar Fairy's job to wander the land in search of people with diabetes. When she found one, she would tap him or her with her magic wand, causing that person's blood sugar to do something particularly wacky. It was deliciously evil. The world of diabetes became chaos. To this day, you can see the results around you. Every once in a while, your blood glucose will do something absolutely crazy. It might shoot up after strenuous exercise, drop after a big meal, or begin to rise soon after a large insulin injection. There seems to be no sense to it!

Of course, the Blood Sugar Fairy doesn't mean to drive you completely crazy; she just enjoys aggravating you. For her, there is no more pleasurable moment than watching someone who is working hard to manage diabetes and is suddenly faced with a surprising result on his or her blood glucose meter: "What? That's impossible! I've eaten the same thing every day this week, and nothing else has changed. There is no way my blood sugar level could suddenly be this high! AARGH!" In recent years, the Blood Sugar Fairy has decided to expand her operation. She now waves her wand at cholesterol levels and blood pressure as well, finding new and even more intriguing ways to make life with diabetes as goofy and inconsistent as possible. Do either of the following scenarios sound familiar?

- Because you have been concerned about your weight, you are carefully following a new meal plan and have increased your exercise. Feeling good about your discipline and progress over the past month, you approach the scale—just as the Blood Sugar Fairy strikes. Surprise, you haven't lost a pound!
- Thanks to a new jogging program, you are finally seeing a significant improvement in your blood glucose levels. What a terrific feeling! But then your hip begins to feel a little funny. Apparently, you've injured it and you will need to stop running for several weeks. The Blood Sugar Fairy strikes again!

DISCOURAGING TIMES

The tale of the Blood Sugar Fairy is a reminder that good actions don't necessarily lead to good results. They often will, but not always. When you are living with diabetes day after day—no matter how diligent your efforts may be—you can be guaranteed that there will be discouraging times. Very discouraging. It cannot be avoided. And how you deal with those moments of aggravation and despair, no matter how big or small they may be, will have a strong impact on your ability to manage your diabetes over the years. Consider the following cases.

Woody and Warren

Neither Woody nor Warren had ever paid much attention to his diabetes. However, after attending a one-day diabetes seminar, they each decided that it was time to take some positive action. Both of them began with small adjustments to the timing of their insulin shots and to their food choices. The results were amazing. Over the next few months, all of their blood glucose readings were consistently below 140 mg/dl. Given their histories, this seemed nothing short of miraculous. Unfortunately, something peculiar began to occur. All of a sudden, their evening blood glucose levels shot up to 250–300 mg/dl, even though there were no changes in their meals or in any other aspect of their lives. After 10 days of this, both were feeling pretty aggravated.

In desperation, Woody decided to make an urgent appointment with a diabetes nurse educator at his local hospital. After careful evaluation, he agreed to adjust his dinnertime insulin and to lengthen his evening walk. This worked out well. Within a few days, his blood glucose levels had fallen back into the 130–140 mg/dl range. Because he was feeling successful, it was easy for Woody to continue with his diabetes care efforts. In contrast, Warren did nothing. As these elevated readings continued, he grew increasingly frustrated, hopeless, and depressed. He felt like smashing his meter. Finally, he decided to cease all blood glucose monitoring, and he gave up even trying to closely manage his diabetes.

Virginia and Rosie

After downplaying the importance of diabetes for many years, Virginia and Rosie had finally decided to get serious about their management of the illness. Both had been diagnosed with type 1 diabetes when they were young children, and it had been several decades since either of them had made much of an effort. In collaboration with their new physicians, Virginia and Rosie worked hard to gain control of their blood glucose. Thanks to their renewed diligence and discipline, their average blood glucose level dropped from 280 mg/dl to 150 mg/dl. Both were delighted. However, tragic events were about to strike.

In Virginia's case, it occurred as she was driving home from work one day. She began to feel a bit sweaty and light-headed and, shortly thereafter, lost consciousness. Next thing she knew, she was in an ambulance on the way to the emergency room. She had suffered a severe hypo-glycemic episode, and her car had been wrecked. Luckily, no one was seriously injured. In Rosie's case, it happened in the middle of the night. She did not have a clear recollection of what occurred, but she knew that she had ended up in a terrible fight with her husband (who was try-ing to get her to drink some juice). And she was eventu-ally taken to the hospital in an ambulance. In all of their years with diabetes, neither Virginia nor Rosie had ever previously experienced such serious hypoglycemia.

Afterward, Virginia was terribly discouraged. She thought to herself, "If this is the sort of thing that happens when you make the effort to take good care of your diabetes, then forget the whole damned thing!" She decided to quit the effort to manage her diabetes intensively, and she allowed her average blood glucose to creep up into the 200–220 mg/dl range. Rosie was also quite upset, but—in contrast to Virginia—she redoubled her efforts. She learned more about hypoglycemia and developed a comprehensive plan for avoiding future episodes (which included evening snacks and more regular blood glucose monitoring at bedtime).

Frank and Herb

Frank and Herb had discovered the joys of exercise. To their mutual delight, they had found that daily exercise (a long walk for Frank, a late afternoon jog for Herb) seemed to curb their appetites, improve their moods, and stabilize their blood glucose. With exercise as a part of their lives, diabetes didn't seem too difficult to handle. They were pleased with their success, and they even boasted to their friends about how well they were managing diabetes. Unfortunately, both Frank and Herb were soon sidetracked.

For several months, Frank had to travel for his job, and then the kids were suddenly sick all the time. With little time for exercise, Frank discovered that he was more nervous, watched more TV, and ate more junk food. His blood glucose began to rise, and he became increasingly disheartened. It felt like everything was starting to unravel.

Herb ran into a similar problem. While out jogging one day, he pulled a muscle quite severely and was forced to limp home. To allow the muscle proper time to heal, his doctor recommended that he stop jogging for a few months. Like Frank, Herb began to feel more edgy. He started snacking more, and he quickly began to put on weight. His blood glucose began to rise too. Greatly discouraged, he wasn't sure what to do.

Although both men were upset by these setbacks, their responses were quite different. After a week of inactivity, Frank decided that he had to find a way to resume exercise. He found a friend who agreed to walk with him at lunchtime on the few days that he was in town each week. In addition, he developed a plan for walking on a regular basis during his travels. Frank was soon back on track. In contrast, Herb sank deeper and deeper into despair. He couldn't think of anything to substitute for his jogging, and his blood glucose and weight kept climbing. By the time his muscle healed, Herb had lost all motivation for exercise and for managing his diabetes.

HOW DOES SHE DO IT?

The Blood Sugar Fairy represents all that is frustrating and discouraging about diabetes. Although good diabetes care almost guarantees good results (excellent blood glucose readings as well as better health in the short and long term), the Blood Sugar Fairy lurks in that one word— "almost." Though you may be putting much time and effort into your diabetes management, there will be occasions when unexpected, weird, or even quite negative results will occur. As you have seen already, these include:

- blood glucose fluctuations that seem to make no sense
- bizarre changes in laboratory values (cholesterol, microalbumin, or glycosylated hemoglobin values that have soared for no earthly reason)
- disappointing changes in your weight
- unforeseen hypoglycemia
- unexpected development of long-term complications (even though you have been managing your diabetes exceedingly well)

Why do these things happen? How does the Blood Sugar Fairy manage to cause such mischief? On many occasions, there is an explanation for the event that can be uncovered through further investigation. Unusual blood glucose readings can result from any of a number of subtle factors, including a fault in your meter, a change in the timing of your diabetes medications, a delayed response to exercise, an unnoticed infection, a change in your meal composition, or—if you take insulin—a problem with your injection site or the potency of your insulin.

On other occasions, there is no apparent explanation for a Blood Sugar Fairy event, at least not with current technology. Thus, it can only be concluded that this unusual occurrence is, simply put, "just one of those things." Indeed, the whole notion of the Blood Sugar Fairy is a polite way of referring to a rarely discussed, though very important aspect of diabetes care. To be blunt, current diabetes treatment, though it is powerful and effective, is still a poor imitation of a fully functioning pancreas. At times, even the very finest of diabetes regimens may not be sufficient to promote good results. Stuff happens.

RESPONDING TO DISCOURAGING EVENTS

Whether there is an underlying explanation or not, most people have a characteristic way of responding to such discouraging events. Some people respond like Warren, Virginia, or Herb—becoming so disheartened that they seem to give up. They have lost the momentum of good diabetes care. Others respond more like Woody, Rosie, or Frank. In the face of discouragement, they somehow tap the inner resources needed to get back on track with their diabetes care. What is going on here? Why were Woody, Rosie, and Frank successful while Warren, Virginia, and Herb were not?

Coping Styles

Researchers have discovered that there are two charac-teristic ways of contending with discouraging events. One approach is known as *emotion-focused coping*. This is when you respond to a difficult occurrence by changing how you think and feel about what has happened. For instance, when someone close to you dies, you might react by thinking about how much you will miss this person, by finding some special, bittersweet way to honor that person's memory, or perhaps even by worrying about your own mortality. Emotion-focused coping is a reasonable and effective approach, especially when there is nothing you can really do to affect the situation.

The second method is *problem-focused coping*. In this approach, you respond by trying to change the situation itself. For instance, when someone close to you is suddenly taken ill, you might respond by collecting more information (asking them to describe what is wrong), calling a doctor, or rushing the sick person to the hospital. Problem-focused coping is the preferred way of reacting when you can have a positive influence on the situation.

Which Style Works?

When the Blood Sugar Fairy strikes, it is easy to assume that there is nothing you can do to repair the situation (after all, you can't even see the Blood Sugar Fairy!). Thus, an emotion-focused coping response would seem most reasonable. In fact, this is exactly what Warren, Virginia, and Herb did. Both Warren and Herb became so discouraged that all they could do was wait and hope for the situation to improve. And Virginia was so focused on her own fear and aggravation that backing away from intensive diabetes management seemed the only answer.

However, the truth is that there is almost always a way to repair what the Blood Sugar Fairy does. Therefore, a problem-solving approach is likely to be more satisfying and effective. Woody, Rosie, and Frank succeeded because they believed that they could *do something* about this discouraging event: Woody saw his nurse educator, Rosie learned more about hypoglycemia, and Frank planned a new exercise program. In all three cases, the path to success was the decision to take thoughtful action.

THE NEXT STEP

Of course, most people will respond to discouragement with an immediate emotional response ("Oh no, not another high blood sugar!"), but the key is what happens next. If you are easily discouraged by diabetes, then you probably continue to react with highly charged feelings ("I hate this! I hate this! I hate this!"), and you never get a chance to focus on resolving the problem. In contrast, the person who uses problem-focused coping will—at least eventually—begin thinking, in a much more dispassionate manner, "Hmmm, now what am I going to do about this?" So overcoming the Blood Sugar Fairy means strengthening your ability to focus on the actual problem and developing strategies for resolving it. How can you do so? There are two major steps to take:

1. Learn more about how to *handle* discouraging diabetes events.
2. Challenge how you *think* about discouraging diabetes events.

Learn More!

By enrolling in a good diabetes education program, you can gain valuable knowledge about how to care for your diabetes and learn more about the necessary problem-solving skills to use during difficult times. Take Virginia, for instance. If she had known that there are many effective strategies for battling severe hypoglycemia (see chapter 17), she might not have felt as hopeless as she did. And if Herb had been more aware of the many different forms of physical exercise as well as the strategies for establishing a new exercise habit (see chapter 8), he might have been more willing to take action.

I have met many people who were at their wit's end, like Woody and Warren, because their blood glucose seemed to bounce around for no earthly reason. Often, closer investigation revealed that variations in the carbohydrate contents of their meals were the major culprit. So they didn't really need to see a psychologist. Instead, they needed to learn about carbohydrate counting! In sum, acquiring knowledge and problem-solving skills can provide you with the hope and confidence that is needed to become a good problem-focused coper. Because diabetes knowledge is constantly expanding, it is important to stay informed as well. Diabetes support groups and relevant magazines (such as *Diabetes Forecast*) are likely to be good resources for you.

Challenge Your Thoughts!

Knowledge can only be helpful if you truly believe that your actions can make a difference. In the face of adversity, those people who feel powerless, that their actions cannot make a difference, are unable to believe that the difficult situation that they face has a solution. Researchers have now found the key to understand and unlock this power of the mind. As it turns out, whether you feel hopeful or hopeless has to do with how you automatically explain to yourself why bad things happen (unfortunately, how you explain to yourself why good things happen doesn't seem to matter very much). This way of thinking is referred to as *explanatory style*. There are three important dimensions of explanatory style to consider. Dr. Martin Seligman, one of the most well-known researchers in this field, refers to them as the three P's: permanence, pervasiveness, and personalization.

Permanence

When a discouraging event occurs, do you automatically think of it as *permanent* or *temporary*? For instance, when struck by severe hypoglycemia, Virginia assumed that this would be an ongoing problem, "Now that I'm managing my blood sugars close to the nondiabetic range, this is certain to happen over and over again." In contrast, Rosie believed that this upsetting event was merely an isolated occurrence. She thought, "Something quite unusual must have happened yesterday for this to have occurred." When his exercise regimen was interrupted, Herb assumed that this disaster would be permanent. He thought "Well, that's it. I'm old and my body's failing, and I will just continue to have injury after injury." However, Frank's assumption was that this interruption would be temporary: "I hate that I am so busy, but I know it won't last for too long."

When you are automatically explaining to yourself that discouraging events are temporary rather than permanent, it colors how you feel about the event. Most importantly, a temporary explanation, like Rosie and Frank made, leads you to believe that you can do something about the situation (change must be possible because this problem is only temporary). A permanent explanation may convince you that you are powerless.

Pervasiveness

When the Blood Sugar Fairy strikes, do you automatically explain it to yourself as something that is universal or specific? Consider the following examples: When his evening blood glucose began to rise, day after day, without any obvious explanation, Warren assumed that these inexplicable changes now infected every aspect of his diabetes care. Discounting the fact that his blood glucose at all other times throughout the day was still below 140 mg/dl, he thought, "Good diabetes care is now impossible. My life will be wrecked." Though Woody was similarly annoyed by the mysterious elevation in blood glucose, his assumption was much more specific: "It now seems impossible to manage my blood sugars during the evening hours. Why is this so different from the rest of the day?" In response to her major hypoglycemic episode, Virginia leaned more toward a generalized explanation of this event, "This will ruin everything, my ability to drive safely and confidently as well as manage my diabetes successfully." However, Rosie's assumption was more specific, "This will wreck my ability to sleep well at night, at least for a while."

When your automatic explanations about discouraging events are specific rather than universal, you will feel more empowered and less hopeless. A specific explanation, such as those Woody and Rosie made, encourages you to believe that your further actions may actually help to resolve the situation. A universal explanation, such as those Warren and Virginia made, leads you to believe that there is nothing that you can do.

Personalization

When a disheartening event takes place, do you automatically assume that the cause is *internal* or *external*? Here are some examples: When his ability to jog was abruptly curtailed, Herb assumed that he was to blame. His immediate thought was, "I am really stupid; I probably could have averted this injury if I had thought about it more." Frank's explanation to himself was more external: "It was the demands of my job and of my family that were to blame. What prevents me from exercising are my circumstances." With his evening blood glucose completely out of whack, Warren assumed that the explanation was internal: "It's all my fault. I must be doing something wrong, but I don't know what it is." In contrast, Woody believed that the cause was external. He thought, "It must be that damned Blood Sugar Fairy. What has she done this time?"

You are more likely to feel powerless when you are making internal rather than external explanations for discouraging events. An internal explanation, such as those Herb and Warren reached, can cause you to feel so bad about yourself that you may be paralyzed into inaction. An external explanation, such as those Frank and Woody reached, prevents you from feeling crippled by self-blame. It allows you to believe that you can fix the problematic situation.

Putting the Three P's Together

If you react to the Blood Sugar Fairy with automatic explanations that tend to be temporary, specific, and external, you are more likely to be problem-focused. In the face of adversity, you will take thoughtful action to resolve the problem. However, if your automatic explanations gravitate toward the permanent, universal, and internal, you are more likely to have an emotion-focused response. When a discouraging event occurs, you are likely to feel powerless and be unable to respond in an effective manner.

Please understand that this has nothing to do with whether you are or are not perceiving the world accurately. For instance, Warren's internal explanation ("It's all my fault. I must be doing something wrong, but I don't know what it is") may be correct, but it still led to him feeling powerless. Frank's temporary explanation ("I hate that I am so busy, but I know it won't last for too long") may be inaccurate, but this belief buoyed his spirits so that he could take action to overcome the problem. Your automatic explanations will influence your ability to respond in an active, problem-solving manner, even though your beliefs may be in error!

YOUR COPING STYLE

How do you explain to yourself why discouraging diabetes events occur? To determine your coping style, please complete Worksheet 18.1 now.

By examining your responses to 1b, 2b, and 3b on this worksheet, you can determine which of the following three styles describes you best.

- If your explanations are typically permanent, universal, and internal, you lean toward a *pessimistic* approach. It is likely that you become overwhelmed when the Blood Sugar Fairy strikes. Problem-focused coping is probably rare for you in these situations.
- If your explanations are typically temporary, specific, and external, you probably recover from any sense of discouragement rather quickly. You lean toward an *optimistic* approach. Problem-focused coping is probably common for you.

■ If the pattern of your explanations does not fall clearly into the optimistic or the pessimistic approach, your style is probably a unique blend of both. You have a *mixed* approach. However, there is likely to be room for improvement. When discouraging events strike, you may not respond as well as you could. Problem-focused coping may be difficult for you.

Now that you have seen how the automatic explanations you make about discouraging events can influence your mood, thoughts, and actions, you can use this information to challenge and change your way of thinking. Of course, if you gravitate toward an optimistic approach (temporary, specific, and external explanations), you may not need to modify your way of explaining events. However, everyone else should please read on!

CHALLENGING YOURSELF

To challenge your habitual way of thinking—never an easy task—it is best to begin and practice with the less difficult moments. The truly discouraging events may be too difficult at first. So, over the next few weeks, whenever a mildly discouraging event occurs, look actively for ways to argue against your characteristic way of explaining what has happened.

If you tend toward permanent explanations, remind yourself that it is just as likely that the repercussions of this event will pass quickly. For instance, when Herb was unable to exercise, you may remember that he concluded, "I'm old and my body's failing, and I will just continue to have injury after injury." Following my suggestion, he argued with himself: "That's ridiculous. I have had very

WORKSHEET 18.1: IDENTIFYING YOUR COPING STYLE

A. *Your past experiences.* Think back on times when something discouraging about your diabetes occurred. These can be minor occurrences (like a surprisingly high blood sugar that occurs one morning) or more major ones (such as a significant weight gain that was not expected). Please select three of the most recent events, then record what happened and how you explained to yourself why this occurred.

Event 1:
What happened?

_____

_____

_____

How did you explain to yourself why this occurred?

_____

_____

_____

Event 2:
What happened?

_____

_____

How did you explain to yourself why this occurred?

_____

_____

_____

Event 3:
What happened?

_____

_____

How did you explain to yourself why this occurred?

_____

_____

_____

WORKSHEET 18.1: IDENTIFYING YOUR COPING STYLE *(continued)*

B. *Rate your explanations.* This may be difficult, but consider how your accounts of the three events fall along the three P's (permanence, pervasiveness, and personalization). Most people will view their explanations as lying halfway between the two extremes of each P, but force yourself to decide whether your explanations tend more toward one end or the other. To gain a more neutral perspective, you might want to enlist the assistance of a friend. Circle the word that best describes your explanation.

1a. Permanence.

Event 1. My account tended toward a (permanent/temporary) explanation.

Event 2. My account tended toward a (permanent/temporary) explanation.

Event 3. My account tended toward a (permanent/temporary) explanation.

1b. Summary.

Of the three accounts, most tended toward (permanent/temporary) explanations.

2a. Pervasiveness.

Event 1. My account tended toward a (universal/specific) explanation.

Event 2. My account tended toward a (universal/specific) explanation.

Event 3. My account tended toward a (universal/specific) explanation.

2b. Summary.

Of the three accounts, most tended toward (universal/specific) explanations.

3a. Personalization.

Event 1. My account tended toward an (internal/external) explanation.

Event 2. My account tended toward an (internal/external) explanation.

Event 3. My account tended toward an (internal/external) explanation.

3b. Summary.

Of the three accounts, most tended toward (internal/external) explanations.

few injuries in the past. There is no evidence that further injuries will occur. It is just as likely that this is a fluke and, with good care, will not occur again."

If you tend toward universal explanations, suggest to yourself that it is always tempting to generalize but a more specific explanation is probably more accurate. For example, Virginia concluded that her hypoglycemic episode and subsequent car crash meant that, "This will ruin everything, my ability to drive safely and confidently as well as manage my diabetes successfully." She challenged this thought in the following manner: "Now wait a minute! Perhaps I am overreacting. Just because I had one serious and quite scary reaction, I shouldn't assume that I will not be able to regain my confidence behind the wheel. Many people with diabetes have had similar experiences and recovered quite nicely. This was certainly an awful episode, but I need to keep it in perspective."

If you tend toward internal explanations, remind yourself that you may be blaming yourself unnecessarily. For instance, when Warren was faced with 10 days of unexplainable high blood glucose levels in the evening, he reasoned, "It's all my fault. I must be doing something wrong, but I don't know what it is." As I recommended, he confronted his typical way of thinking by arguing, "In all honesty, I have no evidence that this is all my fault. There may be other factors at work here that have nothing to do with my self-care actions. I really shouldn't blame myself, at least until I find out more."

A FEW THINGS TO KEEP IN MIND

If you continue to challenge your automatic explanations regularly over a period of several weeks, you will find that it will get easier and easier. Slowly but surely, your sense of hope and confidence in the face of the antics of the Blood Sugar Fairy will build. And as you confront your automatic explanations, please remember three things:

1. **Be kind to yourself.** You live in an imperfect world. The Blood Sugar Fairy exists, and moments of discouragement are likely. Because weird blood glucose levels and other surprising results are certain to occur, at least from time to time, don't be so quick to blame yourself. It might, in fact, be the Blood Sugar Fairy's fault—though I wouldn't recommend that you try that explanation with your physician!

2. **In some cases, the best problem-focused action is no action.** Although you need to believe that your personal actions can make a difference, you also must have the actual skills to accomplish this task. As noted earlier, broad diabetes knowledge and problem-solving skills are essential. As a knowledgeable participant in your own care, you will always respond to the Blood Sugar Fairy's deeds with a thoughtful plan. But this does not necessarily mean that you will take immediate action. For example, what do you do when you see a surprisingly high blood glucose reading in the evening? The best response might be merely to keep good records for several more days to see whether this occurs again over the next few nights or whether some other pattern becomes apparent. In other words, when a confusing result occurs, the best solution is often to avoid an immediate response and, instead, seek to understand what has happened—become more watchful, collect more information, or consult with an expert.

3. **Avoid perfectionism.** You may become discouraged when your expectations are not grounded in reality. If you

feel that all of your blood glucose readings must be perfect, then you are guaranteed to fail. Consider the case of Samantha, a young woman with type 1 diabetes who became burned out on her diabetes because of the terrible disappointment that her blood glucose occasionally rose above 150 mg/dl. To be precise, of the 25–30 blood glucose readings that she would record each week, there were usually two that were higher than 150 mg/dl. Two! What she was ignoring was that her glycated hemoglobin levels had always been between 6.8 and 7.0%, indicating that her overall blood glucose management was excellent. What Samantha needed to learn was that her expectations for blood glucose monitoring were unreasonable, that occasional levels out of her target range were to be expected (the Blood Sugar Fairy at work), and that it was more important to pay attention to her glycated hemoglobin levels. Day-to-day fluctuations will happen, it is the long-term averages that are really important.

So once upon a time, diabetes was the easiest disease in the whole world to manage. Because of the Blood Sugar Fairy, this is no longer true. But this doesn't mean that a happy ending to this fable is impossible. Although weird and wacky occurrences are likely to continue, you can use the strategies presented here to regain a sense of perspective, emotional balance, and humor that will allow you to manage this mischievous little pixie. Who knows? You may even begin to like each other.

Conclusion:
It's Time for Action!

So what have you learned on your journey through this book? You are now likely to:

- Have a clearer perspective on the problem of diabetes burnout.
- Understand that your personal struggle with diabetes does not mean that you are a weak, bad, or unmotivated person.
- Know you are not alone in your struggle.
- Have hope that your physical and emotional health can be improved, motivation can be restored, and burnout can be overcome.
- Realize that the solution to diabetes burnout is to identify and overcome the barriers that may stand in your way.

Instead of feeling overwhelmed and helpless about diabetes, you may have a clearer picture of the personal obstacles that block your path—whether they are social, emotional, environmental, or details of self-care—and have some new ideas about how those barriers can be conquered. With a deeper understanding, you may now be

WORKSHEET 19.1: CREATING A COMPREHENSIVE PLAN FOR ACTION

A. *Your personal barriers.* Of the problems that have been discussed, which do you believe you need to address? Please check any from the following list that you think will require your attention and effort. Since we were not able to cover all of the many possible barriers to good diabetes care, you may be aware of other pressing problems that will need your attention. If so, please include those as well.

Self-Care
___Following a healthy meal plan
___Regular physical activity
___Regular blood sugar monitoring
___Taking medication in a more effective manner
___Other_____

Attitudes and Feelings
___Overcoming depression
___Overcoming fear
___Overcoming denial
___Other_____

Social Relationships
___Obtaining better support from family and friends
___Resolving the problem of the diabetes police
___Improving the relationship with your health care providers
___Other_____

Environmental Stresses
___Reducing life stress
___Managing hypoglycemia more effectively
___Overcoming discouragement (the Blood Sugar Fairy)
___Other_____

B. *Determining your priorities.* If there are only one or two problems that you need to address, then please skip to section C. If you indicated more than two barriers, then it is time to prioritize. What are the top two problems to which you should now give attention? Making this selection may not be easy. Consider that it may be difficult to improve your diabetes self-care unless you are also addressing some of the emotional, social, or environmental obstacles. Most of my patients begin by focusing their attention on one of their problematic self-care behaviors and on one of the emotional, social, or environmental obstacles.

WORKSHEET 19.1: CREATING A COMPREHENSIVE PLAN FOR ACTION (continued)

From the list above, my top two priorities for change are:

1. _____

2. _____

C. *Selecting the actions you will take.* Each chapter includes a recommended set of strategies for overcoming the major diabetes obstacles. Please reexamine the chapters that pertain to your top two priorities for change and select no more than two strategies that you would be willing to try. If you have selected one of the self-care behaviors (except for medication), it might be easier to consult with your completed QuickPlans (see chapter 9). If you have selected an obstacle for which there is no corresponding chapter, please consider whether some of the listed strategies might be of benefit.

1. To address my first priority for change, _____,
   I agree to try the following two strategies:

   a. _____

   _____

   b. _____

   _____

2. To address my second priority for change, _____,
   I agree to try the following two strategies:

   a. _____

   _____

   b. _____

   _____

---

prepared to take action. But how do you know where to begin? Worksheet 19.1 will help you create an action plan.

BABY STEPS

From Worksheet 19.1, you should now have four clear actions that you can take—actions that can help you to begin the process of overcoming diabetes burnout. In reality, there may be a whole slew of problems that you wish to address and strategies that you want to try, but not right now! As was discussed in chapter 9, the best way to begin the process of change is to start with a clear yet limited plan—focusing on goals that are concrete and achievable, being patient with all planned changes, and planning for immediate action. Your selected actions may not be sufficient to completely overcome the particular barriers that they are designed to address, but they can start you moving, step by step, in the right direction. So can you commit to trying these four selected actions within the next week?

If at all possible, do not take these steps alone. Team up with your physician, diabetes educator, family member, friend, or support group. When you have shared your commitment to take some positive action with someone who is rooting for you, your chances of success are magnified.

HOW DO YOU FEEL NOW?

I certainly hope that this book has given you a new way of thinking—and feeling—about diabetes. What do you think? Do you feel any better now about living with diabetes than you did when you began this book? To answer this question, please complete Worksheet 19.2. It's the same as Worksheet 3.1, the questionnaire that you completed at the beginning of chapter 3.

Add up your responses to determine your total score. Then determine which of the four categories represents your score:

- **Not distressed.** Total score is 6–12.
- **Moderately distressed.** Total score is 13–20.
- **Very distressed.** Total score is 21–26.
- **Extremely distressed.** Total score is 27 or higher.

Compare your current score with your score from chapter 3. Perhaps you will find that your total score has dropped.

WORKSHEET 19.2: HOW BURNED OUT ARE YOU?

Directions: In day-to-day life, there may be numerous problems and hassles concerning diabetes and they can vary greatly in severity. Problems may range from minor hassles to major life difficulties. Listed below are several potential problem areas that people with diabetes may experience. Consider the degree to which each of the items may have distressed or bothered you *during the past month* and circle the appropriate number.

Please note that we are asking you to indicate the degree to which each item may be bothering you in your life, NOT whether the item is merely true for you. If you feel that a particular item is not a bother or problem, you would circle 1. If it is very bothersome, you would circle 6.

	Not a problem		Moderate problem		Serious problem	
1. Feeling that diabetes is taking up too much of my mental and physical energy every day.	1	2	3	4	5	6
2. Feeling "burned out" by the constant effort to manage diabetes.	1	2	3	4	5	6
3. Feeling that I am often failing with my diabetes regimen.	1	2	3	4	5	6
4. Feeling that diabetes controls my life.	1	2	3	4	5	6
5. Not feeling motivated to keep up my diabetes self-management.	1	2	3	4	5	6
6. Feeling overwhelmed by my diabetes regimen.	1	2	3	4	5	6

Indeed, you may even find yourself in a new category. Remember that any movement toward less distress, even if you have only shifted from "extremely distressed" to "very distressed," is a positive sign. And if your score has not yet dropped, do not despair. For most people, changes in how you think and feel about diabetes take time.

YOU *CAN* OVERCOME BURNOUT!

The fundamental lesson to remember is that feeling stressed about living with diabetes is normal, feeling at war with diabetes is common, but problematic feelings like these can be conquered. With attention, kindness, and humor, you can overcome diabetes burnout and make peace with diabetes. This is not to suggest that you and diabetes will ever become the best of friends, but you can learn to make room for diabetes in your life. And, as you are certain to discover, this will actually improve the quality, and perhaps even quantity, of your life.

On this journey, you have met a large cast of characters—people who were struggling with diabetes in many different ways as well as those who were tormenting them (the diabetes police, the Blood Sugar Fairy, werewolves, and more). The good news is that all of these folks managed to overcome diabetes burnout and found a way to live in greater harmony with their illness. You can too! And it is my fondest hope that the stories and ideas in this book will help you to achieve that end. I wish you the best of luck along your path.

Index

AMERICAN DIABETES ASSOCIATION
REGIONAL OFFICES

New England Region

7 Washington Square
Albany, NY 12205
518/218-1755
Joyce Waite, Regional Executive Vice
    President

Massachusetts Area Office
617/482-4580

Northern New England Area Office
603/627-9579

Rhode Island Area Office
401/738-6464

Pacific Northwest Region

2480 West 26th Avenue
Suite 120B
Denver, CO 80211
720/855-1102
Mike Van Abel, Regional
    Executive Vice President

Alaska Area Office
907/272-1424

Hawaii Area Office
808/947-5979

Idaho Area Office
208/342-2774

Montana Area Office
406/761-0908

Oregon Area Office
503/736-2770

Washington Area Office
206/352-7950

South Central Region

4425 West Airport Freeway
Suite 130
Irving, TX 75062
972/255-6900
Quincy Neal, Regional Executive
    Vice President

Arkansas Area Office
501/221-7444

Louisiana Area Office
504/831-0278

Northeast Texas/Northern Louisiana
    Area Office
972/392-1181

Oklahoma Area Office
918/492-3839

South Texas Area Office
210/829-1765

West Texas Area Office
806/794-0691

South Coastal Region

1101 North Lake Destiny Road
    Suite 415
Maitland, Florida 32751
407/660-1926
Nancy Carlton, Regional Executive
    Vice President

Atlanta Metro Area Office
404/320-7100

Central Florida Area Office
407/660-1926

Northeast Florida/Southeast Georgia
Area Office
904/703-7200

Northwest Florida/Southern Alabama
Area Office
850/478-5957

Outstate Georgia Area Office
912/353-8110

Southeast Florida Area Office
305/477-8999

Southwest Florida Area Office
813/885-5007

Upstate Alabama Area Office
205/870-5172

Southern Region

2 Hanover Square
434 Fayetteville Square Mall
Suite 1600
Raleigh, NC 27601
919/743-5400
Edward L. Owens, Regional Executive
Vice President

Central North Carolina Area Office
704/373-9111

Eastern North Carolina Area Office
919/743-5400

Greater Hampton Roads Area Office
757/455-6335

Kentucky Area Office
502/452-6072

South Carolina Area Office
803/799-4246

Tennessee Area Office
615/298-3066

Virginia Area Office
804/974-9905

Western Region

10445 Old Placerville Road
Sacramento, CA 95827-2508
916/369-0999
Michael Clinkenbeard, Regional Executive Vice President

Los Angeles Area Office
213/966-2890

Nevada Area Office
702/369-9995

Sacramento Area Office
916/369-0999

San Diego Area Office
619/234-9897

San Francisco Area Office
510/654-4499